Social Aspects of HIV

Volume 8

Since the start of the epidemic, HIV and AIDS have fired the imaginations of social as well as medical and public health scientists. This innovative series of books offers a setting in which to publish the very best of social scientific thinking and research. The Social Aspects of HIV series of books offers readers authoritative introductions and overviews, together with summaries of enduring and cutting edge concerns. The series is international and multidisciplinary in focus, including contributions from psychology, sociology, anthropology, education, economic, political and social theory, and international development. Individual volumes offer scholarly overviews of key topics and concerns but also address 'big issues' relevant to HIV prevention, treatment and care. Sexual and drug-related practices; adherence; disclosure; and stigma and discrimination are among topics focused upon, alongside broader cultural, political and social responses to the epidemic, including globalisation and internationalisation. The political economy of AIDS, links to broader questions of sexual health and rights, and the progressive biomedicalisation of the response, will also be among key issues examined. The series will appeal to those working in public health, health psychology, medical sociology, medical anthropology, health promotion, social work and international development. Individual volumes will be relevant to students, teachers, researchers and practitioners within each of these disciplines as well as program developers and managers working across a variety of contexts.

More information about this series at http://www.springer.com/series/11922

Carmen Logie

Working with Excluded Populations in HIV

Hard to Reach or Out of Sight?

Springer

Carmen Logie
Factor-Inwentash Faculty of Social Work
University of Toronto
Toronto, ON, Canada

ISSN 2509-6559 ISSN 2509-6567 (electronic)
Social Aspects of HIV
ISBN 978-3-030-77047-1 ISBN 978-3-030-77048-8 (eBook)
https://doi.org/10.1007/978-3-030-77048-8

This Springer imprint is published by the registered company Springer Nature Switzerland AG.
The registered company address is: Gewerbestrasse 11, 6330 Cham, Switzerland

For my dearly missed friend and colleague Xolile Sane "Malume" Mabuza, in memory of your joyful, fierce, and courageous activism founding The Rock of Hope in Eswatini and improving the lives of lesbian, gay, bisexual, and transgender persons around the world. Rest in power.

Acknowledgments

The case studies that form the foundation for each chapter in this book were conducted over a 10-year period in various community-based research projects that involved hundreds of participants, peer researchers and peer health workers, research assistants, and colleagues in academia, government, non-government, and inter-governmental organizations. The time, passion, trust, and commitment from each person was key to the research success and to the lessons learned from and about the research process. I am grateful for Peter Aggleton and Richard Parker, series editors, for suggesting this book as a platform to synthesize lessons learned about the concept of "hard to reach" persons across these diverse studies. Their generous, insightful, constructive, and kind feedback was immensely beneficial to my writing process and the final product. Their critical social science research has inspired not only myself but also a generation of scholars to thoughtfully consider the social world in HIV research.

During a sabbatical year in 2020, I was supported by a fellowship at the Brocher Foundation (Switzerland) to focus on writing this book as a visiting researcher. This provided the life altering experience of writing and conducting interviews for each chapter in an office overlooking the Alps and Lake Geneva with the companionship of fellow researchers, and I am forever grateful for the space in which to think and create, the camaraderie for inspiration, and the fresh warm bread each morning. During this time, I was fortunate to have many fruitful discussions on sexual health global research with Manjulaa Narasimhan at the World Health Organization. I was also supported by an Eccles Fellowship at the British Library (United Kingdom) where I was able to read up on seminal HIV activism texts from the 1980s that informed Chap. 5's focus on vernacular knowledge. During this time, I was supported by Ericka Johnson to visit Linkoping University (Sweden) to present findings and engage with scholars in dialogue on community and multi-method storytelling approaches in research. Research on my sabbatical was also supported by a Fulbright Canada Research Chair in Public Health at Johns Hopkins University (United States of America [USA]) that provided opportunities for reading and discussion on global research with socially excluded populations with colleagues and friends in Baltimore, including Stefan Baral, Chris Beyrer, Susan Sherman, Sheree Schwartz, and Andrea Wirtz.

My research program more generally is supported by the Canada Research Chairs Program, Canada Foundation for Innovation, and the Ontario Ministry for Research and Innovation. I am also grateful for the support of faculty colleagues at my home-base at the Factor-Inwentash Faculty of Social Work at the University of Toronto for their continued support and belief in my research, including Dean Voisin. Over the past 15 years, I have benefited from research mentorship that has been invaluable from many, including Mona Loutfy, Peter Newman, and Marion Bogo.

The Jamaican research project described in this book was made possible by funding from the Canadian Institutes of Health Research (CIHR) and the wonderful collaboration with Jamaica AIDS Support for Life (JASL), in particular the Executive Director Kandasi Levermore. Nicolette Richardson (Jones) was an unbelievable force as the research coordinator, and Patrick Lalor, Davina Williams, Tyrone Ellis, Ava Neil, Nicolette Bryan, and Annecka Marshall were key to the project's success. In addition to the participants who shared so much of their lived experience with us, the team of LGBT peer research assistants were essential to the success, as were our collaborators at JFLAG: Jamaica Forum for Lesbians, All-Sexuals and Gays, the Caribbean Vulnerable Communities (CVC), and We Change.

The research in the Northwest Territories, Canada was funded by CIHR and the Social Sciences and Humanities Research Council of Canada (SSHRC). It is based on the outstanding and breathtaking work and vision of Candice Lys, Executive Director and co-founder of Fostering Open eXpression among Youth (FOXY) and Strengths, Masculinities, and Sexual Health (SMASH), the Northern and Indigenous agencies we have been working with for the past several years. Candice, FOXY's peer leaders, co-founder Nancy MacNeill, Setsune (Elder Jane Dragon), Kayley Inuksuk Mackay, and Shira Taylor provided the incredible leadership required for the project's success. In addition, I am grateful for the support of the FOXY board who, in addition to Candice, Nancy, Inuksuk, and myself, also includes leadership from Reneltta Arluk, Sarah Arngna'naaq, and Jay Boast.

The TRANScending Love project with African, Caribbean, and Black transgender women was funded by CIHR and only made possible due to the community activism and leadership of co-principal investigator Yasmeen Persad, a fearless and tireless activist for trans communities. Our research with this project was supported by Wangari Tharao and Denese Frans at Women's Health in Women's Hands Community Health Centre; Shannon Ryan, Dahlak Mary Yehdego, Chris Leonard, and Tatiana Ferguson at Black Coalition for AIDS Prevention (Black CAP); and Monica Forrester at Maggie's Sex Worker Action Project. We were also supported by the 519 Community Center and the Trans Women HIV Research Initiative at Women's College Hospital.

The research project in Eswatini (Swaziland) was funded by the Social Sciences and Humanities Research Council of Canada (SSHRC) and inspired by the chance meeting at the AIDS 2012 conference with Xolile "Malume" Mabuza at a party I attended with Stefan Baral, who I will forever be grateful for introducing us. The

Rock of Hope was an amazing collaborator, led and founded by my dear and deeply missed colleague Malume, and the wonderful team of research assistants include Veli Madau and the academic forte of our colleague Winnie Nhlengethwa at the Southern African Nazarene University made this project a success.

The Grand Challenges Canada and CIHR funded research projects in Haiti were inspired by my colleague and friend CarolAnn Daniel at Adelphi University whose rich experience working in Haiti and qualitative expertise made this project possible. The wonderful collaboration with NEGES Foundation and leadership of Yoleine Gateau, alongside the phenomenal peer health workers, were indispensable to this project's success. I also thank Roro and Jocelyn, alongside the many youth peer leaders.

Scholars, friends, colleagues and activists have inspired and pushed my research and intellectual growth, in addition to each person mentioned above. These include stigma and HIV research colleagues Valerie Earnshaw, Angela Kaida, LaRon Nelson, Laura Nyblade, Amaya Perez-Brumer, Tonia Poteat, Ann Stangl, Janet Turan, and Sheri Weiser. Former and current students I have worked with have also contributed greatly to my learning and growth, particularly Moses Okumu and Ashley Lacombe-Duncan who worked on the Northwest Territories project, and TRANScending Love and Jamaica projects, respectively. My dear friends Jenny Lorito, Danielle Denwood, Eliana Suarez, and Krista Girty have all inspired me to live a meaningful life that extends beyond work.

I also have much gratitude for my family; in particular, my parents Cathleen and Andrew who taught me about hard work, introduced me to travel, and continually encourage me to take time off; my brother Michael and niece Niamh who I only wish lived closer but who know how to enjoy life; and of course, my incredibly supportive, smart, patient, funny, and generous partner Paula who adds laughter, adventure, and joy to the journey. Finally, I must not forget our senior dog Missy and our fleet of motorbikes.

Contents

Chapter 1
Introduction

What do you think of when you hear the term 'hard to reach'? Does a glass on the top shelf in the kitchen come to mind, and needing to bring a step stool over to reach up and grab it? Or perhaps as a researcher, do we think of the challenges we face when people don't show up to our study, and we are left waiting for them? Or maybe we are unable to find the people identified as at 'risk' for HIV who are the focus of our research, making it challenging to meet funding deadlines.

Trying to reach persons who do not seem to want to engage in research, or who we find difficult to locate, is a daunting and at times frustrating endeavour. Why don't people just want to come in and take part in our important study that can potentially benefit them? Is it something about them, maybe their lives are too chaotic? Maybe they do not understand what it is about, and they need more information to make the choice to participate. Or perhaps they have not heard about the study, and we need to figure out how to spread the information to them. Or maybe it is challenging for persons to access the study site due to limited internet or living far away and lacking reliable transportation. All of these scenarios lead us down a path whereby we think that the problem is something that lies outside of ourselves as researchers, and the solution might be to find the metaphorical step stool in order to help people to participate.

But what if instead of looking outside for the problems that create barriers for people to engage with us, we start looking inside ourselves to our own actions and beliefs as researchers? Would we find new perspectives and solutions to thinking about the people researchers find hard to reach? This chapter will provide an overview of the existing literature on people categorized as hard-to-reach and 'hidden'. Specifically, it explores the historical use of these terms and the ways in which they have been applied in HIV research and practice. Attention is paid to how this vocabulary has been used to frame particular communities discussed throughout this book who are disproportionately impacted by HIV.

C. Logie, *Working with Excluded Populations in HIV*, Social Aspects of HIV 8,
https://doi.org/10.1007/978-3-030-77048-8_1

1.1 Historical Use of the Concept 'Hard to Reach'

The concept of people as hard to reach is common in health—particularly HIV—research. For instance, a quick Google Scholar search of the term 'hard to reach' in late 2020 resulted in 4,310,000 hits. Since 2019, there were 67,300 hits. This term has undoubtedly entered the scholarly lexicon. Yet it also remains "contested and ambiguous" with no clear or agreed upon definition (Flanagan & Hancock, 2010). There are many definitions of the word 'hard'. In the Merriam-Webster dictionary, *hard* can be defined as: "difficult to accomplish or resolve: TROUBLESOME", "difficult to comprehend or explain", and "having difficulty in doing something".[1] *Reach* can be defined as "to stretch out", "to touch or grasp by extending a part of the body (such as a hand) or an object", "to extend to", and "encompass, to make an impression on, to communicate with".[2] In fact, as we can see with the MacMillan dictionary thesaurus definition of *'not near and difficult to reach'* the term can mean many things, including distant (remote, far from where you are), isolated, inaccessible and "outermost" (positioned far from the centre).[3]

A literature review reveals the many terms conflated with the notion that persons may be hard to reach, including: vulnerable, marginalized, transient, forgotten, and underserved (Flanagan & Hancock, 2010). Inherent in viewing people as hard to reach is the understanding that they experience social marginalization and stigma that marks them out as different and results in differential access to power and subsequently to resources. Persons marked as hard to reach can also include those who experience challenges accessing health care, such as people with physical, mental, auditory and speech challenges. As a consequence, persons who experience stigma, existing health challenges, and marginalization are often categorized as hard to reach.

Historically, the terms 'hard-to-reach' and 'hidden' populations were not used to describe sub-populations that may be difficult for researchers to access due to stigma, legal confrontations, and physical or other barriers. Persons were instead identified by a particular and specific identity or experience. For example, people who use drugs and sex workers were not referred to as hard-to-reach nor hidden populations but simply as people who use drugs or sex workers. The term hidden population appears to have first emerged in research and literature around 1974 in the UK, in a paper by Bayley who described the pervasive stigmatizing social norms and discriminatory attitudes from police experienced by lesbian, gay and bisexual persons (referred to as 'homosexuals' in the paper) (Bayley, 1974). Bayley coined the term, "hidden homosexuals" to describe people who concealed their sexual orientation from family, friends and especially the police to avoid humiliation, shame and police brutality (Bayley, 1974). In 1976, a paper about the culture and

[1] Definition of hard by Merriam-Webster, https://www.merriam-webster.com/dictionary/hard.

[2] Definition of reach by Merriam-Webster, https://www.merriam-webster.com/dictionary/reach.

[3] Synonym of not near and difficult to reach by MacMillan, https://www.macmillandictionary.com/thesaurus-category/british/not-near-and-difficult-to-reach.

social structure of "gypsies" in America referred to this group as a hidden population because they were nomadic and researchers struggled to reach this population (Morrison & Morrison, 1976).

The term hard to reach became more widely used in the field of social marketing when it was applied to health initiatives for behaviour change (Beder, 1980). Social marketing strategies highlighted the need for creativity and additional funding to reach persons not typically included in standard campaigns. Thus, while in the past people were identified due to socio-demographic characteristics, health and/or social practices, there was a move that appeared to begin in the 1970s to describe persons with the terms hidden and hard to reach. Fast forward to the present day, where there are countless thousands of articles using these terms.

1.1.1 Who Do We Call Hard to Reach?

> Hard-to-reach audiences have been called obstinate, recalcitrant, chronically uninformed, disadvantaged, have-not, illiterate, malfunctional, and information poor. These labels reflect communicators' frustration in trying to reach people unlike themselves and the failure of many campaigns to change high-risk behaviors (Freimuth & Mettger, 1990, p. 323).

The term hard to reach is ambiguous and not well defined and, as described in the above quotation, can reflect our own frustrations of not being able to engage with persons that are in some ways different than ourselves. When researchers and service providers find a population difficult to access for any number of reasons, that population may be labelled as hard to reach. There are numerous ways in which hard to reach persons have been conceptualized. Tourangeau (2014) has disentangled some of the different ways in which people may be experienced as hard to reach: differentiating between hard to sample, hard to identify, hard to find or contact, hard to persuade to participate, and hard to interview. Doherty, Scott, and Kinder (2004) described three hard to reach categories with regards to service delivery: under-represented, including marginalized and socially excluded persons such as ethno-racial minorities and refugees; 'slipping through the net', persons who are invisible, overlooked and/or have constrained agency to voice their priorities, including persons with mental health concerns; and persons who are 'resistant' to services, for multiple reasons, including mistrust, persons targeted by police, and persons who are otherwise disinterested. There are therefore myriad ways that the term hard to reach is applied to understand disengagement and lack of inclusion. Other approaches are detailed below and include (a) sociodemographic, disengagement, and logistic dimensions; (b) dimensions and corresponding tools to identify and work with hard to reach persons; (c) and hidden populations, including persons who do not want to be reached.

1.1.2 Dimensions of Hard to Reach

People may be labelled hard to reach when they share particular socio-demographic characteristics, are disengaged from research and/or health and social services, and when they experience logistic barriers to participation. First, the term hard to reach has been applied across social group memberships. For instance, the label has been applied to: women; lesbian, gay, bisexual, transgender and other sexually and gender diverse persons; ethno-racial minorities; people experiencing homelessness; people who use drugs; sex workers; youth; the elderly; migrants and refugees; people living with HIV; and highly mobile persons (Bacher, Lemcke, Quatember, & Schmich, 2019; Ellard-Gray, Jeffrey, Choubak, & Crann, 2015; Flanagan & Hancock, 2010). A systematic review of 116 studies identified the most commonly referred to hard to reach groups as ethnoracial minorities (40 studies), African American people (19 studies), people who use substances (14 studies), and others more generally labeled vulnerable, minority, or disadvantaged ($n = 11$) (Bonevski et al., 2014). This long list of identities and practices reveal that people belonging to many different sections of society may be labelled hard to reach (e.g., women at large) as well as smaller populations (e.g., sex workers)—revealing the term's lack of specificity. These lists of identities and practices also overlook the intersectionality between social practices and identities, and the implication of holding multiple marginalized identities or practices on being categorized as hard to reach. For instance, is a sex worker who uses drugs easier or harder to reach than non-sex workers who use drugs or sex workers who do not use drugs?

Hard to reach has also been applied to characterize persons who are underserved by social and health services. People's individual attitudes are often considered relevant to disengagement from services. For instance, Brackertz (2007) has described how persons may feel that they are not heard, cared for or about, and/or that services are irrelevant, and therefore may actively decide to disengage. In turn this decision could result in their categorization as hard to reach. Flanagan and Hancock (2010) have thoughtfully discussed the ways that people who do not use services are labelled as hard to reach. Low service uptake could be for many reasons, including persons using non-traditional approaches and resources and in turn not wanting or needing particular services. Although persons who experience greater financial or class privilege may choose not to utilize particular health and social services, or to take part in a research study, they are rarely given the hard to reach label. This suggests that hard to reach is uniquely applied to more marginalized communities and identities experiencing poverty or less class privilege. In this way, hard to reach has become a stigmatizing phrase. Researchers' focus on marginalized populations categorized as hard to reach also reflects a general lack of attention toward persons that are not hard to reach, and who in fact are able and willing to access and participate in research (Katz, Hardy, Firestone, Lofters, & Morton-Ninomiya, 2020). In this way less attention is paid to privilege and power and the ways in which research studies can reproduce existing systems that benefit certain groups while excluding others.

Research studies may not be designed to meet the priorities of the focus population, who in turn make the decision to not participate in research that is not directly relevant or perceived as beneficial. For instance, to avoid duplication of services and to build on existing resources and expertise, agencies may focus on providing a specific service rather than a menu of services (e.g., offering HIV testing alone instead of offering other sexually transmitted infections testing and contraception). This can result in socio-economically and/or geographically marginalized people having to choose where to invest their time or money. Services that are funded may not in fact reflect the priorities of the hard to reach. For instance, a focus of HIV research on LGBTQ communities may look at persons characterized as at high risk for HIV rather than the larger LGBTQ community (Logie & Gibson, 2013). This HIV focus may mean that researchers want to engage LGBTQ persons—but in actuality only include gay and bisexual men and trans women—in HIV prevention and care research. Such an approach actively excludes lesbian, bisexual and queer women from access to community resources, solidarity and social support systems while reinforcing heteronormative beliefs regarding sexual identities and practices among lesbian, bisexual and queer women. Sexually diverse women have unique HIV prevention needs based on sex work engagement, multiple partners, and/or injection drug use, to name a few (Logie, 2015), but these then get ignored. At the same time, an emphasis on HIV biomedical prevention for LGBTQ communities globally can overlook the larger social determinants of health that create elevated exposure to HIV, including family and social exclusion and related mental health challenges, employment discrimination, education discrimination, and housing discrimination. While these larger issues may reflect the priorities of LGBTQ communities, they may often remain beyond the scope of HIV funding envelopes.

Finally, the hard to reach label has been applied to persons who experience logistic barriers to participation. To illustrate this, persons may be classified as hard-to-reach due to their physical/geographic or social locations, including living in remote geographical locations or social elites (Ellard-Gray et al., 2015; Shaghaghi, Bhopal, & Sheikh, 2011). Accessibility barriers may produce hard to reach experiences. Services may be physically inaccessible, via socio-economic concerns such as transport, the lack of childcare, narrow hours, and limited flexibility in one's employment. Other physical access issues include venues that are not wheelchair accessible, or services otherwise not tailored to meet the needs of persons with a disability. Finally, logistic barriers can include a lack of culturally and linguistically relevant resources to facilitate participation. Simply listing these diverse groups of people as hard to reach can overlook the way that positionality is contextually produced, meaning that where people are socially and economically located and how open they are to participating in a service or research project can shift over time and place and reflects larger social and structural inequities.

Social geographies produce particular risks. For instance, research has documented social and health disparities based on public place of sex work (Logie et al., 2020; Logie, White, Galai, Tomko, & Sherman, 2020). Sex workers who work in public settings in contexts where sex work is criminalized experience heightened criminalization and may have to work with a sense of urgency to avoid police arrest, harassment, fines etc. Thus, they have less time and opportunity to engage in research while working outdoors. Conducting research with sex workers who work in outdoor public spaces must therefore consider the elevated violence exposure that persons working in these contexts already experience. Gang boundaries or other territorial markers and community boundaries can also produce barriers for persons from outside to access services. Waiting times can create barriers for all when organizations become busy.

Other logistic social barriers include confidentiality in smaller communities. For instance, in rural and Northern communities in Canada, LGBTQ youth described that there may be no specialized sexual health clinic, and if there was, they may still experience barriers accessing services there as they could know the person working there—they could in fact be a close family friend (Logie et al., 2019). Purchasing condoms and accessing contraception in smaller and rural communities could also mean interfacing with neighbours, family and family friends, and this lack of anonymity produces barriers for accessing services. This has real impacts on health and wellbeing. For instance, there are pervasive STI outbreaks in Northern Canada, and as a result, the public health agencies have had to take creative approaches including expanding services where they offer testing and consider outreach in bars and other public venues. Research in small communities may therefore need to carefully consider and use the most confidential data collection methods, such as individual interviews rather than focus groups, and may need to report socio-demographic characteristics in aggregate form and/or through anonymized quotations to maintain privacy.

1.2 Approaches to Understanding and Reaching the Hard to Reach

Another way that the categories of hard to reach have been understood is in terms of their demographic, cultural, behavioural, attitudinal, and structural dimensions (Brackertz, 2007). Brackertz (2007) developed a tool to identify what characteristics and knowledge are important in understanding who and why persons are hard to reach. This tool describes the importance of examining the demographics (e.g., age, gender, income) of certain populations (such as farmers, youth, Indigenous peoples) to be able to explore group membership dynamics and what activities persons are already engaging in. Cultural factors, including social and institutional exclusion, may highlight the need to work with particular community agencies and within social networks to build connections, including with persons with low literacy, ethno-racially diverse persons, sex workers, and people experiencing homelessness. Attitudes and practices, including mistrust of government and research, and a lack of interest in accessing services or participating in research, underscore the importance of assessing who and what are trusted resources, alternative ways of delivering information and education, social influencers, intervention timing, and outreach strategies. Finally, structural considerations include the timing and location of research activities, the languages and media used for dissemination of study information, and staff and researcher attitudes and competencies. These factors underpin the need to look at alternative ways of communication and delivering information, organizational change needs, and community-academic partnerships that can facilitate engagement with research.

Researchers' focus on persons labelled as hard to reach has largely been on the 'how' to include them in research, with a predominant focus on identifying effective sampling methods (Bacher et al., 2019). Key to such discussion is defining how to sample marginalized populations (Ellard-Gray et al., 2015). For instance, drawbacks and benefits have been proposed regarding various sampling techniques, such as snowball, respondent driven, and quota sampling, to recruit the ostensibly hard to reach person. Starfish sampling, for instance, has been described as a flexible method that integrates both time location sampling (mapping venues to conduct outreach in) and respondent driven sampling (peer referral sampling) for locating transgender men (Raymond, Chen, & McFarland, 2019).

A systematic review (Bonevski et al., 2014) has identified barriers and strategies to sampling, recruitment, data collection, intervention fidelity, and retention. For instance, the sampling barrier of finding it difficult to locate groups of persons could be met with snowball, social networking, and respondent driven sampling. When persons may not want to self-identify, are mobile, and/or when there is no sampling frame the researcher could consider using time-space, targeted, or adaptive sampling, in addition to community-based collaborators. For recruitment barriers of a lack of trust, community-based designs and partnerships are key. Fear of researchers could be mitigated by peer recruitment strategies. Additionally, when persons do not perceive any research participation benefits, other strategies that can be employed include community engagement, offering connections with local resources and services, and shared data ownership. Data collection barriers such as language and literacy may be mitigated by offering the research in multiple languages, multimedia strategies, and interviewer administered (vs. self-administered) data collection. Challenges to intervention fidelity may include the provision of culturally inappropriate services; this challenge can be avoided with sufficient community engagement throughout the study design, adaptation, and pilot-testing processes. Finally, retention barriers may be experienced when working with populations that are very mobile. Researchers can aim to acquire multiple methods of reaching participants as well as any trusted friends. Logistic barriers, such as transport and childcare challenges, can be tackled by offering financial compensation for transport and childcare support and applying tailored and flexible approaches to meeting time and location.

Taken together, this body of work delineates some of the ways in which researchers can identify and tailor steps across the research process to mitigate barriers for persons labelled hard to reach. Such an approach to research should acknowledge and accept there will be additional costs and time in building relationships with communities. The approach requires a long-term perspective that understands relationship building as requiring a significant investment in persons labeled hard to reach.

1.3 Conceptualizing 'Hidden' People

Another term used to describe those that are hard to reach is 'hidden' population (Magnani, Sabin, Saidel, & Heckathorn, 2005; Shaghaghi et al., 2011). The term, *hidden population* is often utilized in research and literature to specifically refer to those who do not want to be found and prefer not to participate in surveillance research due to criminalization and social exclusion. People labelled as hidden may strategically conceal their identity to avoid stigma and criminalization. They may include people who use and sell illicit drugs, LGBTQ persons in contexts with no human rights protections, and/or migrants and persons with precarious immigration status. Criminalization and stigma also create the fear of engaging with health services and research due to surveillance concerns. Sifaneck and Neaigus (2001) describe how there no obvious signs that people who use non-injection heroin are engaged in this practice, and they may in fact decide to sniff rather than inject to "camouflage their membership" regarding heroin use. This camouflaging involves intentional practices to avoid recognition and associated negative social and structural repercussions. In this way, people enact agency to create distance between themselves and researchers in order to prevent experiences that could be negative, such as harm, judgment, and criminalization. For instance, women survivors of violence experience social isolation, constraints regarding communicating about their experiences (including to researchers), and the risk of harms when speaking out about their abuse, and these issues result in limited recognition and record of their experiences (Ellard-Gray et al., 2015). From this perspective, the term hidden can include persons who are socially, legally, economically or otherwise excluded, the systemic structures (legal, policy) and community norms and values that produce this exclusion, and the individual and collective agency that people enact by their decisions to not engage with researchers.

While most of the focus on the hard to reach and hidden comes from the perspective of researchers doing the reaching and searching, less attention is given to the perspectives of the intended participant. How does the focus on reaching and finding the hard to reach or hidden person shape our perspective and reify "genre-structuring constraints (that) limit a speaker's agency" (Black, 2018, p. 85)? A focus on agency can also be applied to better understanding the concept of "hiding" from research and researchers. As Parpart (2013) and others describe, a focus on voice and action in "speaking out" is often framed as emblematic of empowerment, particularly, women's empowerment (Logie & Daniel, 2016; Parpart, 2013). Yet this can obscure the more silent, subtle strategies that are being enacted to navigate inequitable social and structural contexts and to negotiate power in relationships. Seen from this perspective, guarding the secrecy and privacy of one's lived experiences by hiding them from researchers is not simply a passive, powerless position; rather, it can reveal a survival strategy that is carefully managed.

Persons who are hidden, an adjective defined by Merriam-Webster as "being out of sight or not readily apparent", may in fact be assessing ways to *hide*, a verb they define as "to conceal for shelter or protection". Silence and secrecy have a long history in shaping survival strategies for marginalized groups, including in conflict situations (Parpart, 2013). Instead of perceiving hiding as passive and problematic, it may at times be the opposite for persons who experience social, economic, and/or political precarity and who subsequently have an understandable fear of surveillance. This "politics of silence" has informed the silence survival strategies of multiple populations impacted by HIV, including lesbian, gay, bisexual and transgender persons, sex workers, people who use drugs, people who experienced sexual violence in conflict, as well as people living with HIV. For instance, persons may conceal their HIV positive serostatus to reduce the likelihood of rejection, blame, discrimination and, in some cases, the harms of criminalization. Disclosure in research settings, as in social life, requires cost-benefit analyses and this decision making is an example of enacting agency even in rights-constrained situations.

1.4 Examples from Research with People Labelled Hard to Reach

Groups commonly labelled as hard to reach in public health, and particularly HIV research where they are disproportionately represented, include people who use drugs, sex workers, gay men, and migrant or mobile populations. Lin, Zhang, He, and Zhao's (2019) review describes the term hard to reach as inclusive of persons who may engage in practices, and/or hold identities or other characteristics, that are stigmatized by community members and healthcare providers (Lin et al., 2019). These groups are often reported as more challenging to locate than other populations who typically access health care, and therefore require more time and resources for recruitment and retention. As Magnani et al. (2005) describe it, "Because public health resources are scarce, surveillance has traditionally targeted the 'low hanging fruit' (i.e., the most easily accessed populations) for HIV surveillance" (Magnani et al., 2005, p. S68).

People who use drugs have often been labelled as hidden and hard to reach in HIV and other health research. An ethnographic approach to engaging people who were non-injection ('sniffer') heroin users has discussed the microenvironments in which people who use drugs were living, and pointed to the need for researchers to acquire both access to these settings and an understanding of the languages prevalent within them (Sifaneck & Neaigus, 2001). Ethnographic methods may help to uncover the worldview of people who use drugs and their practices, both of which will enhance access to this hidden population and can be used to inform the development of appropriate and relevant research and sampling approaches. This ethnographic study aimed to understand day-to-day life and the way that drug use was embedded to provide a thick description of person's lives:

> For many users, the non-injected use of heroin was not the central focus of their self-identity, just as, for the social drinker, a glass or two of wine in an appropriate setting and at an appropriate time is an acceptable activity which does not define the user's identity. If anything, non-injecting heroin users wished to distance themselves from the heroin scene (Sifaneck & Neaigus, 2001, p. 523).

The above quotation signals a few considerations regarding persons characterized as hidden. First, the identity that the researcher is privileging in research may not be a central identity embraced by a potential participant. Second, an identity may be stigmatized and steeped within in-group social hierarchies, in this case, non-injection vs. injection heroin use. Thus, persons may want to distance themselves from the stigma associated with the practice of heroin use, and more specifically from others they perceive to be lower down in the social hierarchy due to particular injection practices. These socio-cultural identities may be unknown to the researcher unless they first conduct ethnographic or similar investigations to understand contexts and cultures within micro-environments. This in-depth knowledge was used to inform research methods spanning sampling, recruiting and screening grounded in "ethnographic accessing" (Sifaneck & Neaigus, 2001, p. 528). Interestingly, this study points not only to the need to identify persons who are not always easily identified, but also to understand the changing context of a phenomenon such as heroin use so as to include persons who reflect a spectrum of experiences. This spectrum necessitates different approaches to recruitment, including developing an "ethnographic" presence in neighbourhoods.

Ethnographic snowball sampling has also been described as an approach that aims to engage persons not just for financial compensation but also because of their socio-political interests. Targeted canvassing informed by ethnography could include a spectrum of locales, including media, community, bars and clubs, and street-based approaches. For instance, in studies with people who inject drugs, such a non-judgmental approach to recruitment does not assume that drug use unproblematically equals identity. Another study with people who used non-injection heroin sent birthday cards with redeemable gift certificates as a means to stay connected and build trust. The authors described how "the cards reflected personalized attention and to a certain extent a sense of empathy from the research staff that many respondents had not previously experienced" (Cepeda & Valdez, 2010, p. 708). Research approaches such as this that combine contextual knowledge and engagement of field workers who have shared social and life experiences with the focus population have facilitated high levels of participant retention.

Gay, bisexual and other sexually diverse men have also been described as hard to reach in HIV research, in part due to the pervasive stigma and discrimination experienced by LGBTQ persons in global settings (Fredriksen-Goldsen & Kim, 2017; Guillory et al., 2018; Prescott et al., 2016). Same sex sexual practices remain criminalized in 70 countries, exacerbating stigmatizing social, community and familial norms and contributing to health inequities and research exclusion (International Lesbian, Gay, Bisexual, Trans and Intersex Association, 2019). Yet this idea that gay, bisexual and other sexually diverse men are inherently hard to reach is challenged by the explosion of social media and subsequent harnessing of this as a recruitment method. For instance, Martinez et al.'s (2014) study used social media to reach Latino gay couples in the USA and discussed that this was in fact not a hard to reach population (Martinez et al., 2014). A systematic review of social media interventions to reach gay, bisexual and sexually diverse men that included eighteen studies from high income countries, and eight from middle-income countries (none from low-income countries), reported that social media platforms (e.g. Facebook) and dating apps (e.g. Grindr) were associated with increased HIV testing uptake (Cao et al., 2017).

Baral et al. (2018) were able to create population size estimations of gay, bisexual and other sexually diverse men from Sub-Saharan Africa (South Africa, Ghana, Nigeria, Senegal, Cote d'Ivoire, Mauritania, Gambia) as well as Lebanon, Thailand, Malaysia, Brazil, Ukraine and the USA using data from the Hornet Gay Social Network and Facebook. What was novel about their study was that it showed that estimates of the numbers of gay, bisexual and other sexually diverse men were higher when using social media approaches to estimation than had previously been reported by UNAIDS. The underestimation of the existence and 'reachability' of gay, bisexual and MSM required thoughtful and collaborative research with local community agencies and responded to calls by advocate groups that required data to acquire funding to support gay, bisexual and other sexually diverse men in programs and resources.

This example illustrates the importance of questioning even well-resourced and reputable sources, such as UNAIDS, when it comes to reaching marginalized populations such as gay and bisexual men. This is not, however, to gloss over the many challenges for survival experienced by gay, bisexual and other sexually diverse men across the world. For instance, conservative social norms, stigma, and criminalization of same-sex sexual practices result in HIV prevention campaigns that largely exclude gay and bisexual men, and present profound barriers to participating in HIV testing and care (Mozafari & Mayer, 2017). There remains limited knowledge about the HIV prevention needs of gay, bisexual and MSM in certain contexts, such as in the Arab states, due to the hiddenness of this population. This contextual and shifting heterogeneity of who is hard to reach, by whom, and when, should be considered as this term cannot be applied to persons such as LGBTQ communities in a static or universal manner.

1.5 What Are the Implications of Using the Term Hard to Reach?

Application of a single term to individuals and populations such as hard to reach or hidden implies that there is a thread of homogeneity within distinct sub-populations which does not necessarily exist (Brackertz, 2007; Shaghaghi et al., 2011). For example, sex workers who use drugs and experience homelessness can be considered as belonging to several hard to reach populations that can be difficult for researchers to connect with. However, from an intercategorical, intersectionality perspective these sub-populations of sex workers, people who use drugs, and persons experiencing homelessness, can all have distinct lived experiences of opportunity and oppression that intersect with race, socioeconomic status, immigration status, ability, among other identities and experiences (McCall, 2008). There is also complexity within communities, and a person who uses drugs may not necessarily be homeless, and a sex worker may not necessarily use drugs. Applying an intracategorical perspective encourages further exploration of these issues.

For instance, an intracategorical, intersectional lens might explore shared and different experiences among sex workers based on gender, homelessness, sexual orientation, ethno-racial identity, among other social identities and practices. Among gay men, it may be easier for researchers to access gay men in the USA than in some other settings due to contextual differences in rights afforded to LGBTQ persons, signaling intracategorical differences within populations of gay men. Even in a study with transgender communities in the same country (the USA), persons who are more likely to be accessed in person than online include trans persons who are women, persons of colour, and have lower incomes and educational levels (Reisner et al., 2013). These examples underscore heterogeneity within groups of sex workers, gay men, and trans women, based on intersecting identities that shape access to and engagement with research studies.

Studies also point to the salience of intercategorical approaches to understanding the role of gender in shaping different lived experiences and HIV prevention needs among women and men engaged in sex work. For instance, HIV prevalence was significantly higher among cisgender men sex workers compared to cisgender women sex workers in Jamaica (Logie, Wang, Lalor, Williams, & Levermore, 2021). Among urban refugee adolescents and youth in Uganda, young women engaged in transactional sex had increased condom efficacy and condom use compared with young women not engaged in transactional sex (Logie et al., 2020). This signals how young women engaged in transactional sex had increased sexual agency. Yet the situation was reversed among young men: those engaged in transactional sex had 68% lower odds of HIV testing than their counterparts not engaged in transactional sex. Intercategorical and/or intracategorical intersectional approaches can therefore be applied to how we understand who exactly is hard to reach, and why, and to better understand the diversity within and between communities.

1.5.1 Whose Perspective Is Included/Excluded?

In their study of persons in the voluntary sector working with persons categorized as hard to reach, Flanagan and Hancock (2010) report that professionals and service users within the sector dislike the term. In fact, participants explained that they and the services they offer were often what was hardest to reach. Services and research can be exclusionary when they are not designed in ways that meet the needs of the intendent participants. For instance, one service user described "I am not 'hard to reach', generally people don't know how to reach me" (Flanagan & Hancock, 2010, p. 5). The term hard to reach also fails to reflect the larger social and institutional contexts that produce barriers for people to reach services, resources, or studies. The term may also overlook whether or not the person being labelled hard to reach actually identifies themselves as such. Indeed, the person you want to take part in a study may not consider themselves at all hard to reach, hence this term can be experienced as stigmatizing (Willis, Smith, Shariff-Marco, & English, 2014).

1.5.2 Whose Responsibility Is It to Reach Who?

> It makes it sound like the fault of the non service-user 'you are hard to reach'—like they are sat up on a shelf and we have got to lure them down with biscuits, or something .... actually, if you just got a ladder and sat next to them that would be fine (Flanagan & Hancock, 2010, p. 4).

This quotation above suggests that blame may be attributed to the service user for the challenges that researchers have in reaching them. It also places responsibility on the researcher to move position and change their stance. In effect, researchers should move closer to the people and communities that they want to connect with, rather than waiting for persons to come to them. This signals who holds power in the relationship: researchers and others in institutional positions of power can dictate the space(s) they want the hard to reach person to occupy, revealing the expectation that the other person will move and in effect change their position. This occludes reflection on power relationships. For instance, researchers can reflect on the connections they have with the communities they want to reach, explore how their own objectives reflect community objectives, and engage community members in developing research objectives and methods that will translate to community benefits. Are the challenges researchers experiencing finding persons due to their biases toward communities labelled hard to reach? Self-reflection on these biases can also create space to better understand the values, preferences and perspectives of the individuals and communities researchers are trying to reach.

1.6 Understanding the Hard to Reach Through the Lens of the Epistemology of Ignorance

> Ignorance should not be theorized as a simple omission or gap but is, in many cases, an active production. Ignorance is frequently constructed and actively preserved, and is linked to issues of cognitive authority, doubt, trust, silencing, and uncertainty (Tuana, 2004, p. 195).

Framing persons as hard to reach is also grounded in the notion that those doing the reaching lack the knowledge of how to find persons. This lack of knowledge can be explored by applying conceptualizations from the epistemology of ignorance that elucidates the multiple ways in which ignorance can be understood.

1.6.1 Ignorance as Propositional

The standard and accepted understanding of ignorance is that it comprises a lack of knowledge or belief—yet this approach to ignorance is contested (El Kassar, 2018; Peels, 2010). This position is also considered the '*propositional conception of ignorance*.' (El Kassar, 2018, p. 301). Peels (2010) describes how doxastic attitudes include a belief or disbelief that something is true, or a suspension of judgment due to not considering something or holding no particular belief regarding its truth. He further describes how doxastic attitudes can be both *occurrent,* which refers to considerations, thoughts or reflections on a belief, or *latent*, when the belief is present without having been actively considered, thought or reflected on (Peels, 2010). This propositional approach conceptualizes four types of ignorance: someone disbelieves something that is true (disbelieving ignorance); someone does not have a judgment on something that is true (suspending ignorance); someone has never considered something that is true, but would not believe it (conditional disbelieving ignorance); and someone has never considered something that is true, but would suspend judgment if they considered it (conditional suspending ignorance) (Peels, 2010). Suspending judgment may be rooted in *deep ignorance* (a lack of knowledge or cognitive abilities) that differs from *evidential ignorance* (a lack of sufficient evidence to form a belief).

This propositional perspective on ignorance considers both the person and their context, as well as facts and subject matter. For instance, a heart surgeon who does not know how to perform heart surgery could be considered ignorant, whereas a secondary school student without heart surgery knowledge would not be considered so. The HIV researcher engaged in social science research, for instance, could be considered ignorant for being unable to engage marginalized communities in HIV research. Ignorance can be used as an excuse for moral responsibility, whereby lack of knowledge could result in harm (Peels, 2010). When persons have conducted insufficient investigations that result in a lack of discovery and action they may be considered to blame for their ignorance (Smith, 1983). Ignorance has also been described as an excuse for incorrect and false beliefs.

Tactics to address the problem of the hard to reach in HIV research, and that focus on strategies of how to find persons, are premised on the idea that the challenge lies in the researchers' ignorance due to a lack of knowledge about the people they are trying to reach. From this perspective, the solution is to learn and acquire knowledge of where to find these hard to reach persons, and how to entice them to engage in research. Engaging the hard to reach thereby becomes a project of acquiring the specialized knowledge and skills that will be adequate for engaging participants. The researcher's role in this approach to ignorance is to learn more about the hard to reach person in order to develop better strategies to find them. This propositional approach to ignorance informs many of the methods-focused textbooks and articles for researchers providing knowledge and tactics to find and engage hard to reach persons.

1.6.2 Ignorance as Agential

A second approach to the epistemology of ignorance, rooted in feminist and critical race theory, approaches ignorance as an active engagement in practices that uphold false outlooks. This approach to ignorance perceives ignorance as not only missing knowledge but as a form of epistemic injustice that is actively developed and maintained (El Kassar, 2018; Tuana, 2004). Oppression is often cloaked by ignorance, as power shapes what is known and subsequently what is not known by constructing particular topics, people, and issues as having value, function and importance. Ignorance also fluctuates over time and, as Tuana (2004) describes it, sometimes ignorance practices have the consequence of 'unlearning' a knowledge domain. While some areas and populations are missing from formal knowledge systems, others have been unlearned, and the important consideration is who this ignorance benefits and who it disadvantages.

Tuana (2004) traces the epistemology of ignorance regarding women's sexuality and pleasure using the lens of intersecting power, knowledge and ignorance over time. Specifically, she demonstrates the politics of ignorance over women's sexual pleasure with a case study of female genitalia, and the ways in which current medical science privileges knowledge of men's sexual organs. She details a history of the clitoris, from sixteenth century knowledge of women's sexual organs and pleasure to the twentieth century omission from medical texts, followed by feminist movements in the 1970s and 1980s that provided more detailed imagery of sexual organs and discussion of sexual pleasure (Tuana, 2004). Tuana (2004) situates inequitable knowledge production regarding female sexual organs and women's pleasure as the products of a politics of ignorance that is rooted in patriarchy and compulsory heterosexuality, which focuses on (heterosexual) male pleasure and sees women's sexual organs as existing primarily for reproduction. The same socio-political forces that obscured women's sexual organs also constructed same-sex sexual practices and attractions as deviant. This example reveals the ways in which socio-political power produces knowledge and ignorance and how "what we attend to and what we ignore are often complexly interwoven with values and politics" (Tuana, 2004, p. 219). Notably feminist movements were stimulated to produce detailed knowledge of women's sexual organs and pleasure in response to their exclusion from medical texts. This example of the ways in which knowledge of women's sexual organs was omitted from medical science, but then reintroduced by feminist movements, reveals the ways in which 'lost knowledge' can be reclaimed, the political nature of medical knowledge and its flipside of ignorance regarding socially marginalized bodies' sexual organs and pleasures, and the important role of activism and social movements in challenging epistemologies of ignorance.

Another example of oppressive systems of ignorance includes white ignorance, whereby whiteness shapes false beliefs systems regarding the existence of Black and other people of colour and ignorance of racial injustice and its impacts (Mills, 2007, 2015). For instance, persons can create a worldview that ignores evidence and can refuse to consider perspectives and lived experiences different from their own. Ignoring evidence moves beyond propositional evidence, which is a lack of knowledge, to epistemic practices that reproduce willful ignorance. In characterizing white ignorance Mills (2007) invites the reader to:

> Imagine an ignorance that resists.
>
> Imagine an ignorance that fights back.
>
> Imagine an ignorance militant, aggressive, not to be intimidated, an ignorance that is active, dynamic, that refuses to quietly—not at all confined to the illiterate and uneducated but propagated at the highest levels of the land, indeed presenting itself unblushingly as knowledge. (p. 13)

Mills describes how white racism causes ignorance toward Black persons and other persons of colour and in turn produces an epistemic asymmetry where ignorance is not reciprocal. Black persons and other persons of colour are required to learn about white people and cultures due to white supremacy, whereas the reverse is not true. In fact, white people may live out their lives in North America and other white dominated places without ever needing to learn about Black people's cultures and lived experiences. In this way, Mills (2007) explains how:

> Often for their very survival, blacks have been forced to become lay anthropologists, studying the strange culture, customs, and mind-set of the "white tribe" that has such frightening power over them, that in certain time periods can even determine their life or death on a whim ... What people of color quickly come to see—in a sense, the primary epistemic principle of the racialized social epistemology of which they are the object—is that they are not seen at all. (p. 18)

Knowledge of women's sexual pleasure, same-sex sexual practices, and Black and other persons of colour (and those at the intersection of these experiences) is produced in ways that simultaneously construct persons as being both at risk for HIV and hard to reach. A second example of oppressive systems of ignorance lies in epistemic practices of arrogance, laziness and closed-mindedness that produce a form of *active ignorance*. Medina has described: "active ignorance is an ignorance that occurs with the active participation of the subject and with a battery of defense mechanisms, an ignorance that is not easy to undo and correct, for this requires retraining—the reconfiguration of epistemic attitudes and habits—as well as social change" (Medina, 2013, p. 39). This approach to ignorance implies attitudes and habits that extend beyond a lack of knowledge as understood as propositional ignorance. El Kassar (2018) describes this as an *agential conception of ignorance* which assumes that that persons are epistemic agents who both produce and reproduce ignorance, with this (re)production being rooted in maintaining socio-political inequities (El Kassar, 2018).

1.6.3 Ignorance as Structural

A third approach to ignorance conceptualized by Alcoff (2007) is to conceive it as a *structural, substantive epistemic practice* that involves practices by individuals, societies and structures that construct beliefs (Alcoff, 2007). This approach posits that ignorance practices are produced and reproduced in structural and social contexts, including ignorance that is willfully promulgated to maintain socially acceptable faulty beliefs. This structural conception of ignorance approaches ignorance as a negative practice that is formed by, and maintains, social and structural inequities. For instance, ignorance services functions such as reproducing and sustaining privilege, traditional values and belief systems, and maintaining stereotypes.

Structural approaches to ignorance as a 'bad practice' also point to strategic ignorance. For instance, from 1996 to 2001 Purdue Pharma produced ignorance of the potentially addictive nature of OxyContin by systematically misrepresenting the risk of addiction and widely recommending its use for pain relief (Van Zee, 2009). Purdue later pleaded guilty to these criminal charges for false claims that OxyContin was linked to lower addiction risks and abuse than other opioid painkillers, and was charged $634 million USD. Yet by this time Purdue had widely influenced physicians to prescribe opioids more liberally with an aggressive national marketing campaign that also targeted particular physicians and US regions with the highest opioid prescribing patterns (Van Zee, 2009). Not only were healthcare professionals engaged in all-expenses paid symposia, and provided branded promotional products ranging from hats, toys and music, they were also hired for speaker's bureaux (Van Zee, 2009). In this example, social and structural forces in Big Pharma and healthcare actively produced ignorance regarding OxyContin's addictive properties as a substantive epistemic practice.

Tobacco manufacturers have also claimed ignorance of health risks of tobacco's links to cancer in order to avoid lawsuits. McGoey (2012) discusses this in the context of ignorance as an organizational resource, particularly regarding how drug regulation involves arguments over preserving the least knowledge of safety concerns regarding drugs in order to avoid liability (McGoey, 2012). Knowledge, and knowing what to know, are socio-political. Using the case example of the drug Ketek, an antibiotic drug produced by Sanofi-Aventis and associated with liver failure, multiple practices in testing and licensing were used to cultivate ignorance, including concealing data, suppressing staff resistance, and ignoring the limits of evaluating drug-related harms (McGoey, 2012). This deliberate muddying and disconnection from information result in what McGoey refers to as *strategic ignorance* that serves to acquire and retain resources, reject liability in the case of problems, and maintain expert control (McGoey, 2012). Labelling persons as hard to reach may also be part of the strategic ignorance practised by researchers to avoid responsibility for failing to provide research aligned with a community's interest. This can reinforce the researcher's expert position, allowing them to continue to use the same research strategies instead of propelling them to learn new approaches to connecting with communities. For instance, acquiring and retaining research funding by ignoring the hard to reach may make it easier to reach objectives, whether these are retention in longitudinal studies or meeting sample size requirements. Such funding objectives may be easier to reach with persons who are not labelled hard to reach.

Heimer discussed the ways in which HIV clinics have used strategic ignorance (Heimer, 2012). Awkward knowledge is kept hidden by confining its accessibility, often in organizational and regulatory files that produce an illusion of knowledge, and by strategically separating facts using organizational roles and/or boundaries (Heimer, 2012). The first example provided in this case study of HIV clinics is *sequestered knowledge* that refers to unsettling information, or inconvenient facts, that are rendered inert by being hidden in bureaucratic paperwork. The second example is *distributed ignorance*, produced when persons focus on their own work, what they know, and do not acquire group knowledge of what others are working on in their agency (Heimer, 2012). Distributed ignorance can be both unintentional, due to a lack of time or resources to synthesize the information, and/or purposeful, by keeping types and sources of information separated. HIV clinics are an institutional example of the nexus of multiple interests—public health programs, research, and donor expectations—that have roots in power imbalances between expert providers and clients and do not always consider social and structural inequities.

Part of the role of HIV clinical research sites is recruitment and research ethics protocol management, and informed consent processes for clinical trials may be a culturally variable ritual (Heimer, 2012). For instance, in the USA potential participants are expected to read and sign a consent form, often while listening to highlights of the study as described by the researcher. In countries such as Uganda, however, participants typically have the form read aloud to them by the researcher who offers to respond to queries and questions. The researcher may also return at a second point in time to read the form aloud again to potential participants and may then test participants on the content of the informed consent forms. These differences in informed consent procedures symbolize different concerns regarding knowledge of consent processes, as well as literacy levels that could be reviewed by monitoring boards.

Underlying concerns about research participation are ideas about coercion, and it is arguable whether research with marginalized persons can be non-coercive when persons are participating for benefits such as honoraria, drug treatment, access to health care, and the perceived benefits of care. Yet not perceiving people as able to provide informed consent can also be patronizing and overlook agency and the cost/benefit decision making that most people engage in daily. The research ethics process involves extensive documentation, often in language that can be challenging for participants to understand. This process is largely developed by research ethics boards and researchers, often with little engagement of the persons they are hoping to recruit. Heimer has described:

> ... we do not have adequate ways of talking about risk, harm and the uncomfortable choices people confront, allowing people to choose to remain ignorant about some things (the ambiguities of consent) allows them to reduce ignorance about others (which therapies work). In this regime, a proper research subject is one who has signed a consent form and that signed form papers over any ambiguities (Heimer, 2012, p. 24).

The need to align with HIV funding expectations may create additional pressures, particularly when the funder requires bans on sexual and reproductive health and rights services, such as focusing on heterosexual and cisgender persons, abstinence, and the exclusion of sex workers. For instance, the global gag rule and PEPFAR have encouraged the USA to fund sexual and reproductive health practices that are not evidence-based, including abstinence and abortion bans (Mavodza, Goldman, & Cooper, 2019; Singh & Karim, 2017). This can place agencies who provide non-abstinence HIV prevention messaging and resources, and/or abortion services, in an awkward position—particularly in the Global South where service providers may rely on donors from the USA for much of their funding—to try to serve their clients and their clients' needs while not 'breaking rules'. This leads to sequestering information and performing rituals to satisfy donors, while simultaneously working in the backstage beyond the public gaze to manage the uncomfortable information.

Part of the challenge in HIV research and practice lies in managing physical and social side effects. For instance, the side effects of antiretroviral therapy may make it difficult to maintain a regular regime, particularly if food and/or housing is insecure. This becomes more problematic in contexts of HIV criminalization that require an undetectable HIV viral load. For instance, in Canada, a person currently needs to have an undetectable viral load and use a condom if they do not want to disclose their HIV positive serostatus without possible criminal charges, even in the absence of HIV transmission. Yet the social side effects of disclosure of HIV include stigma and discrimination that can impact on family, intimate partner and friend relationships, and on employment, among other negative repercussions. Thus, HIV researchers focused on HIV testing and/or adherence need to balance intended and unintended benefits and side effects. This can lead to muddying, overlooking, ignoring and concealing such physical and social side effects in order to retain participants and meet funder targets.

In a similar way, a funding focus on reaching HIV biomedical outcomes may overlook the mental and emotional priorities of participants. This may lead to distributed ignorance in choices regarding what research is focused on (and whose interests are and are not reflected in research), what programs are delivered, and what medication/services people are offered. What happens when persons access drugs such as PrEP that are not covered by a health plan at a clinical trial and the trial finishes? Researchers and clinicians may need to remain ignorant about what happens post-trial in order to acquire funding, fulfil the immediate need to conduct the study and produce scientific knowledge, as well as offer the immediate benefits of HIV prevention, in the case of PrEP. Distributed ignorance reflects a lack of comprehensive, holistic perspectives and may seem inevitable due to the division of organizational labour and power. For instance, researchers may not have the power or funds to offer PrEP following a study so may instead focus solely on the immediate study period. Agencies also have boundaries within which they operate, constraining where in the environment they can meet their clients, such as home, school and work versus the research office. Knowledge of anticipated and unanticipated side effects can decrease distributed ignorance, but at times—such as those discussed above with reference to pharmaceutical and tobacco companies—institutions with a vested financial interest may instead prefer to keep some facts 'inert'.

1.6.4 An Integrated Approach to the Epistemology of Ignorance

El Kassar has proposed a conceptualization of the epistemology of ignorance that seeks to integrate elements from propositional, active and structural approaches discussed above (El Kassar, 2018). While it may often be the case that persons lack knowledge or have mistaken beliefs (reflecting a propositional approach to ignorance), feminist and critical race frameworks signal the importance of *agential approaches to agency*. Agential approaches remind us that people hold agency and power over their epistemic practices. The idea of *epistemic agency* includes the ways that people acquire, store, process, share, and evaluate knowledge and beliefs (Goldberg, 2014). An integrated approach to ignorance can reflect these myriad perspectives: there is need for knowledge acquisition, people are agentic and hold power over their knowledge practices, and structural and social forces and dynamics (re)produce false knowledge. By simultaneously considering these approaches to ignorance as interconnected and legitimate, propositional, agential, and structural conceptions become "interlocking components of ignorance that react just like in a chemical reaction between elements" (El Kassar, 2018, p. 305). Holding these components together results in an integrated conceptualization of the epistemology of ignorance that considers the ways in which ignorance is constructed by both a person's beliefs (either not knowing and/or believing) as well as their epistemic attitudes that may include virtues such as open-mindedness and curiosity and vices, such as closed-mindedness and arrogance. Such a perspective acknowledges the individual's agency in their own ignorance and provides space for examining the social and political factors that shape epistemic attitudes. Within this approach, our attitudes are in fact part of our ignorance—and are not just caused by ignorance. This integrated approach to ignorance is also congruent with sociology of practice and sociology of memory perspectives that view knowledge as always incomplete, selective, and amenable to manipulation to meet personal and structural demands (McGoey, 2012). A focus on ignorance also builds on notions of *undone science,* whereby research questions may be overlooked to due political backlash, and *negative knowledge*, referring to research domains that persons have no interest or motivation to further explore (Frickel et al., 2010).

1.7 HIV Research and the Epistemology of Ignorance

Our attitudes toward how and what we know may underpin our ignorance about how to reach certain persons. For instance, although two researchers may be deeply ignorant (from a propositional approach to ignorance) about the barriers that transgender persons face in accessing health systems to receive services, their epistemic attitudes may differ. One may be open-minded, wanting to learn and increase their understanding of the barriers and the potential ways they can reduce barriers and increase research participation. The other researcher, however, may be closed-minded and disbelieving of these barriers, choosing to hold on to false ideas about the problem lying within the individual and their attitudes toward research. Beliefs and knowledge therefore have different consequences based on one's epistemic attitudes. From the perspective that persons can be responsible for maintaining their own ignorance regardless of the reasons behind this practice, there is an onus on researchers to consider their approach to acquiring, processing and assessing their own knowledge and beliefs regarding persons labelled hard to reach. There is also a need to examine institutional practices across education, political, religious, legal, and healthcare spheres. Specifically, researchers can reduce their culpability for addressing ignorance by calling on *knowledge alibis*, described as:

> The ability to defend one's ignorance by mobilizing the ignorance of higher-placed experts. A curious feature of knowledge alibis is that experts who should know something are particularly useful for not knowing it. This is because their expertise helps to legitimate claims that a phenomenon is impossible to know, rather than simply unknowable by the unenlightened. If the experts didn't know it, nobody could (McGoey, 2012, p. 564).

How then are the systems that HIV researchers live and work in implicated in producing knowledge and ignorance regarding persons labelled as hard to reach? This introduction has outlined the contested nature of the ways in which we understand and label persons as hard to reach, as well as approaches to solving the problem of connecting with persons who are categorized as such. In HIV research, the hard to reach are often constructed as populations that need to be identified for inclusion into research. There has been less focus, however, on the role of HIV researchers in producing or transforming the contexts whereby people find it challenging to participate in research and/or decide to hide from and avoid inclusion in research studies. HIV researchers need to invest more time and care in building relationships with the persons they wish to conduct research with and for; these relationships may help researchers to connect with communities they may otherwise find it difficult to engage in research. A key question to be asked in this respect is what are our connections with and to the populations we want to work with, and how do our research processes meaningfully engage and centre the people we want to study? The term hard to reach implicitly focuses on the difficulty researchers experience finding persons to participate in research studies, casting the researcher's gaze outward to the problem they must solve in order to find their ideal participants.

However, epistemology of ignorance perspectives towards the framing of the hard to reach support a critical examination of this idea that researchers simply do not know how to reach certain persons and communities. Researchers' lack of information about marginalized communities does not exist in a vacuum, rather it is co-produced alongside attitudes towards knowledge, such as humility, open-mindedness or arrogance and close-mindedness. Our knowledge is also shaped by privilege and power. Researchers may consider what knowledge they acquired about the people they want to reach in their education, and personal and professional lives. In another reflection, researchers can consider why or why not they have close relationships and knowledge about the people they want to include in research studies. Within this reflection, researchers can examine what actions they have taken to build relationships and generate new understandings about communities labelled hard to reach. Finally, researchers can think about the institutions they find themselves embedded within, such as higher education, healthcare, and legal systems, and how these systems have historically and currently treated persons considered hard to reach.

The label hard to reach calls to mind the problems that researchers may be having in locating persons and communities. Have researchers also documented in a similar manner the strengths, community cohesion, collective agency, resilience and resistance of persons categorized as hard to reach? Intersectional frameworks are rooted in community care, solidarity, collective action for liberation, and recognize the wisdom and experience passed on across generations (Collective, 1981). Strengths-based researchers can amplify the assets and strengths that exist among communities who are problematized by the hard to reach label; for instance, researchers developed the #BlackGirlMagic framework to build on Black women's strengths (Walton & Oyewuwo-Gassikia, 2017) and strengths-based case management to support people living with HIV who use drugs (Kral et al., 2018). Resilience frameworks can also identify the processes that foster wellness among groups including Indigenous youth (Njeze, Bird-Naytowhow, Pearl, & Hatala, 2020), gay and bisexual men (Herrick, Stall, Goldhammer, Egan, & Mayer, 2014), transgender women (Sun, Anderson, Mayer, Kuhn, & Klein, 2019), and sex workers (Burnes, Long, & Schept, 2012). Together, these examples signal the potential of a strengths-based research lens to produce new knowledge of the capacity, wisdom, and potential in persons and communities categorized as hard to reach.

1.8 Rethinking 'Hard to Reach'

Building on these ideas, this book aims to rethink who is hard to reach—is it researchers or is it communities that researchers struggle to engage with? In answering this question, the book will share case examples from community-based research conducted with and for lesbian, gay, bisexual and transgender (LGBT) youth in Jamaica, Indigenous youth in Northern Canada, African Caribbean and Black transgender women in urban Canada, LGBTQ persons in Eswatini, and internally displaced women in post-earthquake Haiti. Rather than offering a 'how to' approach, the book will instead reflect on approaches and perspectives for researchers to consider when building meaningful and reciprocal relationships with socially, economically and/or politically excluded persons and communities.

Chapters signal the need for attention to five key social factors when developing approaches for meaningful research engagement: context, cultural humility, critical hope, imagination, and love. Individually and together, these factors can inform how nations, institutions, communities, and individuals may work together to address HIV in a sustainable and impactful way. Chapters each include three components. First, each chapter begins with a description of the research study drawn upon and some personal reflection on my own learning moments. Second, the chapter includes a conversation between myself and a researcher central to each community-based project. In this conversation the co-researcher reflects on their experience of the research project, the concept of the community we worked with as being labelled hard to reach, and recommendations for future research. The conversations were digitally recorded and transcribed verbatim, and subsequently shared with the co-researcher who could make edits and additions to better reflect their perspective and experiences on the research study. This reflective process of conversation embraces a solidarity approach to research, whereby instead of writing about the project from a distance, all of the field notes (our recorded conversation, my personal reflection, the chapter as a whole) "become group documents, subject to discussion and mutual comment and learning" (Glesne, 2007). The approach also reflects a collaborative witnessing approach, whereby I engage in co-storytelling in each chapter to bear witness not only to my own memories of what happened, but also the co-researcher's memories and reflection on my interpretation of events (Rawicki Jerry, 2013). This reflects approaches from *friendship as method* that draw on personal and social experiences as well as emotional connections, in this case between myself and the co-researcher (Tillmann-Healy, 2003). Friendship as method aligns with critical feminist resistance to the idea that research can ever be value-free and involves multi-voice reflections that add "emotional and relational layers to ... intellectual pursuits." (p. 734) (Tillmann-Healy, 2003). While not strictly adhering to a friendship as method approach, each of the studies involved multi-year time commitments that resulted in long-lasting relationships with co-researchers and opportunities for retrospection on the research journey. I also strive for radical reciprocity throughout the book, a tenet of friendship as method, that shifts the gaze from observing "them" to observing "us" (Tillmann-Healy, 2003,

p. 735). The third and final section of each chapter includes historic and current conceptualizations of each facilitating factor and how it may be relevant to working with socially excluded persons in HIV research.

A collaborative approach to remembering and interpreting lessons learned from research may help the reader to grasp the essence of the study beyond a singular perspective:

> . . . knowledge production is an intentional process . . . we are neither cameras, passively capturing a snapshot of the social landscape, nor mirrors, reflecting back on objective reality. Instead we are active agents seeking to learn about our world through each piece of data that we collect (Suzuki, Ahluwalia, Arora, & Mattis, 2007, p. 323).

The process of writing this book has elicited curiosity, caring, and compassion about co-researchers' experiences and perspectives, in turn deepening these relationships and my own learning and growth as a researcher. I hope that together these multiple perspectives can challenge the notion that persons are ever hard to reach, amplify our shared humanity, and strengthen our commitment to social justice.

References

Alcoff, L. M. (2007). Epistemologies of ignorance: Three types. In S. Shannon & N. Tuana (Eds.), *Race and epistemologies of ignorance* (pp. 39–58). New York: State University of New York.

Bacher, J., Lemcke, J., Quatember, A., & Schmich, P. (2019). *Probability and nonprobability sampling: Representative surveys of hard-to-reach and hard-to-ask populations. Current surveys between the poles of theory and practice. Survey methods: Insights from the field.* Retreived from https://surveyinsights.org/?p=12070. https://doi.org/10.13094/SMIF-2019-00018

Baral, S., Turner, R. M., Lyons, C. E., Howell, S., Honermann, B., Garner, A., Iii, R. H., Diouf, D., Ayala, G., Sullivan, P. S., & Millett, G. (2018). Population size estimation of gay and bisexual men and other men who have sex with men using social media-based platforms. *JMIR Public Health and Surveillance, 4*(1), e15.

Bayley, B. H. (1974). The policeman and the homosexual: Encounters and attitudes. *New Sociology, 1*(4), 18–52.

Beder, H. W. (1980). Reaching the hard-to-reach adult through effective marketing. *New Directions for Adult and Continuing Education, 1980*(8), 11–26.

Black, S. P. (2018). The ethics and aesthetics of care. *Annual Review of Anthropology, 47*(1), 79–95.

Bonevski, B., Randell, M., Paul, C., Chapman, K., Twyman, L., Bryant, J., Brozek, I., & Hughes, C. (2014). Reaching the hard-to-reach: A systematic review of strategies for improving health and medical research with socially disadvantaged groups. *BMC Medical Research Methodology, 14*(1), 42.

Brackertz, N. (2007). *Who is hard to reach and why?* ISR Working Paper. Swinburne University of Technology.

Burnes, T. R., Long, S. L., & Schept, R. A. (2012). A resilience-based lens of sex work: Implications for professional psychologists. *Professional Psychology: Research and Practice, 43*(2), 137–144.

Cao, B., Gupta, S., Wang, J., Hightow-Weidman, L. B., Muessig, K. E., Tang, W., Pan, S., Pendse, R., & Tucker, J. D. (2017). Social media interventions to promote HIV testing, linkage, adherence, and retention: Systematic review and meta-analysis. *Journal of Medical Internet Research, 19*(11), e394.

Cepeda, A., & Valdez, A. (2010). Ethnographic strategies in the tracking and retention of street-recruited community-based samples of substance using hidden populations in longitudinal studies. *Substance Use and Misuse, 45*(5), 700–716.

Collective, C. R. (1981). A black feminist statement. In C. Moraga & G. E. Andaluza (Eds.), *This bridge called my back: Writings by radical women of color* (pp. 234–244). Berkely, CA: Third Women Press.

Doherty, P. A., Scott, A., & Kinder, K. (2004). *Delivering services to hard to reach families in on track areas: Definition, consultation and needs assessment*. Home Office Development and Practice Report, 15.

El Kassar, N. (2018). What ignorance really is. Examining the foundations of epistemology of ignorance. *Social Epistemology, 32*(5), 300–310.

Ellard-Gray, A., Jeffrey, N. K., Choubak, M., & Crann, S. E. (2015). Finding the hidden participant: Solutions for recruiting hidden, hard-to-reach, and vulnerable populations. *International Journal of Qualitative Methods, 14*(5), 160940691562142.

Flanagan, S. M., & Hancock, B. (2010). "Reaching the hard to reach" - Lessons learned from the VCS (voluntary and community Sector). A qualitative study. *BMC Health Services Research, 10*.

Fredriksen-Goldsen, K. I., & Kim, H.-J. (2017). The science of conducting research with LGBT older adults - An introduction to aging with pride: National Health, Aging, and Sexuality/Gender Study (NHAS). *The Gerontologist, 57*(suppl_1), S1–S14.

Freimuth, V. S., & Mettger, W. (1990). Is there a hard-to-reach audience? *Public Health Reports, 105*(3), 232–238.

Frickel, S., Gibbon, S., Howard, J., Kempner, J., Ottinger, G., & Hess, D. J. (2010). Undone science: Charting social movement and civil society challenges to research agenda setting. *Science, Technology & Human Values, 35*(4), 444–473.

Glesne, C. (2007). Research as solidarity. In M. Denzin & N. Giardina (Eds.), *Ethical futures in qualitative research* (pp. 169–178). Left Coast Press.

Goldberg, S. (2014). *A proposed research program for social epistemology*. Social Epistemology and Epistemic Agency, November.

Guillory, J., Wiant, K. F., Farrelly, M., Fiacco, L., Alam, I., Hoffman, L., Crankshaw, E., Delahanty, J., & Alexander, T. N. (2018). Recruiting hard-to-reach populations for survey research: Using Facebook and Instagram advertisements and in-person intercept in LGBT bars and nightclubs to recruit LGBT young adults. *Journal of Medical Internet Research, 20* (6), e197.

Heimer, C. A. (2012). Inert facts and the illusion of knowledge: Strategic uses of ignorance in HIV clinics. *Economy and Society, 41*(1), 17–41.

Herrick, A. L., Stall, R., Goldhammer, H., Egan, J. E., & Mayer, K. H. (2014). Resilience as a research framework and as a cornerstone of prevention research for gay and bisexual men: Theory and evidence. *AIDS and Behavior, 18*(1), 1–9.

Katz, A. S., Hardy, B. J., Firestone, M., Lofters, A., & Morton-Ninomiya, M. E. (2020). Vagueness, power and public health: Use of 'vulnerable' in public health literature. *Critical Public Health, 30*(5), 601–611.

Kral, A. H., Lambdin, B. H., Comfort, M., Powers, C., Cheng, H., Lopez, A. M., Murdoch, R. O., Neilands, T. B., & Lorvick, J. (2018). A strengths-based case management intervention to reduce HIV viral load among people who use drugs. *AIDS and Behavior, 22*(1), 146–153.

Lin, D., Zhang, C. Y., He, Z. K., & Zhao, X. D. (2019). How does hard-to-reach status affect antiretroviral therapy adherence in the HIV-infected population? Results from a meta-analysis of observational studies. *BMC Public Health, 19*(1), 1–13.

Logie, C. H. (2015). (Where) do queer women belong? Theorizing intersectional and compulsory heterosexism in HIV research. *Critical Public Health, 25*(5), 527–538.

Logie, C. H., & Daniel, C. (2016). "My body is mine": Qualitatively exploring agency among internally displaced women participants in a small-group intervention in Leogane, Haiti. *Global Public Health, 11*(1–2), 122–134.

Logie, C. H., & Gibson, M. F. (2013). A mark that is no mark? Queer women and violence in HIV discourse. *Culture, Health and Sexuality, 15*(1), 29–43.

Logie, C., Lys, C., Dias, L., Schott, N., Zouboules, M. R., MacNeill, N., & Mackay, K. (2019). "Automatic assumption of your gender, sexuality and sexual practices is also discrimination": Exploring sexual healthcare experiences and recommendations among sexually and gender diverse persons in Arctic Canada. *Health & Social Care in the Community, 27.*

Logie, C. H., Okumu, M., Mwima, S., Hakiza, R., Abela, H., Kyambadde, P., Helen, C., Okumu, M., Mwima, S., Hakiza, R., Mwima, S., Hakiza, R., & Abela, H. (2020). Gender, transactional sex, and HIV prevention cascade engagement among urban refugee and displaced adolescents and youth in Kampala, Uganda. AIDS Care, *0*(0), 1–7.

Logie, C. H., Wang, Y., Lalor, P., Williams, D., & Levermore, K. (2021). Pre and post-exposure prophylaxis awareness and acceptability among sex workers in jamaica: A cross-sectional study. *AIDS and Behavior, 25*(2), 330–343.

Logie, C. H., Wang, Y., Lalor, P., Williams, D., Levermore, K., & Sherman, S. G. (2020). Exploring associations between place of sex work and HIV vulnerabilities among sex workers in Jamaica. *International Journal of STD and AIDS,* 31(12), 1186-1194.

Logie, C. H., White, R. H., Galai, N., Tomko, C., & Sherman, S. G. (2020). Brief report: Longitudinal associations between place of sex work and client condom coercion among sex workers in Baltimore, Maryland. *Journal of Acquired Immune Deficiency Syndromes (1999), 85* (5), 579–583.

Magnani, R., Sabin, K., Saidel, T., & Heckathorn, D. (2005). Review of sampling hard-to-reach and hidden populations for HIV surveillance. *AIDS (London, England), 19(Suppl 2)*, S67–S72.

Martinez, O., Wu, E., Shultz, A. Z., Capote, J., López Rios, J., Sandfort, T., Manusov, J., Ovejero, H., Carballo-Dieguez, A., Chavez Baray, S., Moya, E., López Matos, J., DelaCruz, J. J., Remien, R. H., & Rhodes, S. D. (2014). Still a hard-to-reach population? Using social media to recruit latino gay couples for an HIV Intervention Adaptation Study. *Journal of Medical Internet Research, 16*(4).

Mavodza, C., Goldman, R., & Cooper, B. (2019). The impacts of the global gag rule on global health: A scoping review. *Global Health Research and Policy, 4.*

McCall, L. (2008). The complexity of intersectionality. *Intersectionality and Beyond: Law, Power and the Politics of Location, 30*(3), 49–76.

McGoey, L. (2012). The logic of strategic ignorance. *The British Journal of Sociology, 63*(3), 533–576.

Medina, J. (2013). The epistemology of resistance: gender and racial oppression, epistemic injustice, and the social imagination. In The epistemology of resistance: Gender and racial oppression, epistemic injustice, and the social imagination. Oxford University Press.

Mills, C. (2007). White ignorance. In S. Sullivan & N. Tuana (Eds.), *Race and epistemologies of ignorance* (pp. 11–38). State University of New York Press.

Mills, C. W. (2015). Global white ignorance. In *Routledge international handbook of ignorance studies.* Oxon, United Kingdom.

Morrison, P., & Morrison, P. (1976). Gypsies: The hidden Americans. *Scientific American, 234*(1), 131–134.

Mozafari, M., & Mayer, K. H. (2017). Social change and HIV in Iran: Reaching hidden populations. *The Lancet HIV, 4*(7), e282–e283.

Njeze, C., Bird-Naytowhow, K., Pearl, T., & Hatala, A. R. (2020). Intersectionality of resilience: A strengths-based case study approach with indigenous youth in an urban Canadian context. *Qualitative Health Research, 30*(13), 2001–2018.

Parpart, J. (2013). Choosing silence: Rethinking voice, agency and women's empowerment. In R. Ryan-Flood & R. Gill (Eds.), *Secrecy and silence in the research process: Feminist reflections* (pp. 15-29). New York, NY: Routledge.

Peels, R. (2010). What is ignorance? *Philosophia, 38*(1), 57–67.

Prescott, T. L., Phillips, G., II, DuBois, L. Z., Bull, S. S., Mustanski, B., & Ybarra, M. L. (2016). Reaching adolescent gay, bisexual, and queer men online: Development and refinement of a national recruitment strategy. *Journal of Medical Internet Research, 18*(8), e200.

International Lesbian, Gay, Bisexual, Trans and Intersex Association (ILGA): Lucas Ramon Medos. (2019). State-Sponsored Homophobia 2019. Geneva; ILGA World.

Ellis, C., & Rawicki, J. (2013). Collaborative witnessing of survival during the holocaust: An exemplar of relational autoethnography. *Qualitative Inquiry, 19*(5), 366–380.

Raymond, H. F., Chen, Y.-H., & McFarland, W. (2019). "Starfish sampling": A novel, hybrid approach to recruiting hidden populations. *Journal of Urban Health, 96*(1), 55–62.

Reisner, S. L., Conron, K., Scout, N., Mimiaga, M. J., Haneuse, S., & Austin, S. B. (2013). Comparing in-person and online survey respondents in the U.S. national transgender discrimination survey: Implications for transgender health research. *LGBT Health, 1*(2), 98–106.

Shaghaghi, A., Bhopal, R. S., & Sheikh, A. (2011). Approaches to recruiting 'hard-to-reach' populations into re-search: A review of the literature. *Health Promotion Perspectives, 1*(2), 86–94.

Sifaneck, S. J., & Neaigus, A. (2001). The ethnographic accessing, sampling and screening of hidden populations: Heroin sniffers in New York City. *Addiction Research and Theory, 9*(6), 519–543.

Singh, J. A., & Karim, S. S. A. (2017). Trump's "global gag rule": Implications for human rights and global health. *The Lancet Global Health, 5*(4), e387–e389.

Smith, H. (1983). Culpable ignorance. *The Philosophical Review, 92*(4), 543–571.

Sun, C. J., Anderson, K. M., Mayer, L., Kuhn, T., & Klein, C. H. (2019). Findings from formative research to develop a strength-based HIV prevention and sexual health promotion mHealth intervention for transgender women. *Transgender Health, 4*(1), 350–358.

Suzuki, L. A., Ahluwalia, M. K., Arora, A. K., & Mattis, J. S. (2007). The pond you fish in determines the fish you catch: Exploring strategies for qualitative data collection. *The Counseling Psychologist, 35*(2), 295–327.

Tillmann-Healy, L. M. (2003). Friendship as method. *Qualitative Inquiry, 9*(5), 729–774.

Tourangeau, R. (2014). Defining hard-to-survey populations. In R. Tourangeau, B. Edwards, T. P. Johnson, K. M. Wolter, & N. Bates (Eds.), *Hard-to-survey populations* (pp. 3–20). Cambridge University Press.

Tuana, N. (2004). Coming to understand: Orgasm and the epistemology of ignorance. *Hypatia, 19* (1), 194–232.

Van Zee, A. (2009). The promotion and marketing of oxycontin: Commercial triumph, public health tragedy. *American Journal of Public Health, 99*(2), 221–227.

Walton, Q. L., & Oyewuwo-Gassikia, O. B. (2017). The case for #BlackGirlMagic: Application of a strengths-based, intersectional practice framework for working with black women with depression. *Affilia - Journal of Women and Social Work, 32*(4), 461–475.

Willis, G. B., Smith, T. W., Shariff-Marco, S., & English, N. (2014). Overview of the special issue on surveying the hard-to-reach. *Journal of Official Statistics, 30*(2), 171–176.

Chapter 2
Context and Storytelling

This chapter explores ideas about context and storytelling in research through the example of a community-based research study conducted with LGBT[1] youth in Jamaica. The first part includes a reflection on the research process and key learning moments. Following this there is a conversation with the research coordinator, Nicolette Richardson (née Jones), who worked with the community partner Jamaica AIDS Support for Life in Kingston, Jamaica. The final section of this chapter explores the wider literature on context and storytelling, and its relevance to understanding research with LGBT persons in rights-constrained contexts such as Jamaica.

2.1 Reflections on Learning Moments from Working with LGBT Persons in Jamaica

As a doctoral student, in 2009 I was invited to a conference in Kingston, Jamaica to present findings from some research on stigma. While there, I met with a number of people from a community-based AIDS service organization called Jamaica AIDS Support for Life (JASL). We immediately connected over our shared interest in the experiences of stigma among LGBT persons. After many months of conversation, we developed a grant proposal in 2012 to understand LGBT young persons' (aged 18–24) experiences of stigma and how these experiences shaped HIV prevention and access to care access. The first phase, started in 2013, involved qualitative methods and aimed to elicit first-hand perspectives on stigma with focus groups and in-depth interviews. A subsequent quantitative phase from 2014 to 2016 involved a

[1]The acronym LGBT here is used, rather than LGBTQ, as no participants in our study identified as queer.

C. Logie, *Working with Excluded Populations in HIV*, Social Aspects of HIV 8,
https://doi.org/10.1007/978-3-030-77048-8_2

cross-sectional survey in which we offered HIV and syphilis testing and treatment through JASL's clinics.

Learning moments throughout this study helped me to reconsider the meaning of concepts such as 'liberation' for LGBT persons, provided a new perspective on stereotypes of Jamaica, allowed me to become a more flexible and responsive researcher, and helped me to understand what translating research into action can look like. The first of these learning moments happened quite soon after the study had begun. I went to Kingston to train the peer researchers who were to help with recruitment and data collection. As focus group moderation is challenging and requires careful management of group dynamics, we decided I would co-facilitate the focus groups with the research coordinator Nicolette and a peer researcher. The first focus group was with young gay and bisexual men. During this focus group there were several occasions when I found myself surprised by the stories that were shared. Among stories of violence, rejection and hardship, one young man described his mother buying him a mannequin during secondary school on which to practice hairdressing—considered a feminine occupation. He subsequently received emotional and financial support from his family to pursue this vocation. Another young man, who described living in a low-income neighbourhood he referred to as a ghetto, reported that he could be gay and look as feminine as he wanted to with no harmful repercussions so long as he did not bring any men home with him. These narratives show pockets of acceptance in what has been called one of the most homophobic places on earth (Jackson, 2015), and a setting in which same-sex sexual practices remain criminalized (Ramon Mendos, 2019).

I had expected that all of the participants would want same sex sexual practices decriminalized, based on reading human rights journals and LGBT advocacy materials. Yet when I asked about this, one of the young gay men discussed how he did not want the focus to be on decriminalization as there would be backlash and associated violence targeting LGBT persons. Before decriminalization, he explained, we needed to change the hearts and minds of people in the community, the media, church, and politicians in order for legal change to help bring about any real social change. Participants recounted events from a planned Pride gathering the prior year. The hardware stores had sold out of machetes, and even some of the focus group participants went to purchase a machete or brought their own to line the streets where the pride march was planned. If they had not done this, they might have been assumed to be gay.

This sparked a conversation about what pride can look like for LGBT persons in rights-constrained environments such as Jamaica. Gay and bisexual men participants described how they did not need or necessarily strive for what was happening with LGBT persons in North America. For instance, participants explained that they did not feel the need to walk down the street holding their partner's hand as 'this was Jamaica' and these practices were not congruent with the local context. Participants reported feeling that they would be happy if they were able to live lives free of violence and discreetly engage in intimate relationships. Afterwards when I came back to Canada and discussed how my assumptions of LGBT youth priorities in Jamaica (what I had assumed would include decriminalization, Pride celebrations, and public displays of affection) were challenged after listening to lived experiences I was met with disbelief from both academics and non-academics. How could persons not want decriminalization—could it be that informants did not really understand the importance of structural-level change? Yet young LGBT persons identified the need to invest in and prioritize grassroots, community-based change in social norms and attitudes toward LGBT persons *first* in order to create and sustain legal change. And this local knowledge of what needed to happen to spark sustained social change has also been demonstrated to be true in countries like India, that saw initial legal changes regarding decriminalization of same sex sexual practices later overturned when there was insufficient support at the community-level among the general public. I was struck by the way in which I had unconsciously accepted the idea that North America had the template of what LGBT persons might want in Jamaica. I had overlooked the range of possibilities for LGBT liberation, and had not considered how things might unfold differently in a more collectivist society.

Several years into our study in Jamaica, I was in Kingston during an International Day Against Homophobia, Transphobia and Biphobia (IDAHOT) celebration where the annual focus was on love. The celebration required pre-registration and was held in an upscale hotel to increase security. The speakers' narratives discussed how LGBT people across the Caribbean maintained long, loving intimate partnerships and included conversations with same-gender couples. This approach—focusing on love and learning from the lived experiences of LGBT persons in the Caribbean in long-term partnerships—was appreciated and embraced for its contextual relevance. Prevailing notions of LGBT liberation from the West may advocate for a rights-based approach as opposed to an approach centered on learning from nurturing and loving partnerships. A rights-based approach focused on modelling pathways to LGBT liberation in North America might aim to hold Pride celebrations—which are now increasingly happening in Jamaica. Yet these celebrations are not without risks, as evidenced in the 2017 death of Dexter Pottinger who was described as the then 'face' of Jamaica's LGBT pride. Dexter was a Jamaican fashion designer and queer activist. He had a central role in organizing Jamaica's Pride Week, and was murdered in his home later that year.[2] The person charged with his murder pleaded guilty using a 'gay panic defense'[3] predicated on the idea that a victim provoked their own murder by making sexual advances to someone of the same gender.[4]

Participant narratives revealed a complex story that moves us beyond simple notions of Jamaica being a homophobic country. The most common response in academic and non-academic circles when I discuss my research in Jamaica is 'Jamaica is so homophobic!' In the course of the study, we did in fact collect stories of extreme violence; stigma; familial, religious and community exclusion; and

---

[2]https://www.nylon.com/articles/dexter-pottinger-jamaican-lgbtq-activist-murdered.

[3]https://www.gaystarnews.com/article/man-uses-gay-panic-defense-in-murder-of-jamaican-fashion-designer/.

[4]https://theconversation.com/i-track-murder-cases-that-use-the-gay-panic-defense-a-controversial-practice-banned-in-9-states-129973.

mistreatment by healthcare providers, educators and family members. At the same time, however, participants' narratives spoke of family members who were accepting and supportive, of LGBT communities that continued to expand and advocate, and of strategies LGBT people employed to navigate their identities and relationships within the Jamaican context.

The stories people tell can have real consequences. In Kingston, many transgender (trans) women focus group participants lived outside under a bridge in an area called the 'gully'. We provided them with transport to the focus group location as they did not feel safe on public transport. A short while after our focus group took place, a documentary was produced by non-Jamaicans about trans women that lived in the gully in Kingston. Colleagues on the ground and peer researchers reported that the backlash to this documentary was one of violence—including the state-sponsored removal of trans women from this location. While a bridge may not be ideal housing, it does provide shelter from the elements. Our conversations with trans women revealed that many had moved to living in the bushes beside a parking lot. That parking lot was subsequently bulldozed. Trans community members then squatted in a vacant house that was later set on fire. While anecdotal, these stories from persons on the ground signal the potential for well-meaning non-Jamaican activists to prioritize issues and actions (such as a producing a documentary) that may have harmful repercussions.

Another learning moment concerned the way in which research could inform timely responses to community needs. Focus groups and interviews with trans women revealed extreme poverty—including challenges acquiring and retaining employment and housing due to stigma. JASL used these qualitative findings to apply for and receive funding to provide support to trans women. This was an immediate and swift action to mobilize research to benefit the community. Simultaneously, they realized the need for transgender competency training for all JASL staff in order to provide an affirming space for transgender persons. To address this need JASL hired trans persons from a community agency to train their staff in three clinics. This commitment to translate research findings into immediate action, and to change workplace norms and attitudes to better serve a marginalized group, reflected flexibility and responsiveness.

Another example of responsiveness lay in changing the scope and focus of the study. While originally planned as a single-site study in Kingston, JASL requested that we expand work to their other clinic locations in Ocho Rios and Montego Bay. In addition to expanding locations, there was so much interest from gay, bisexual and other sexually diverse men that we doubled the sample size. However, recruitment was much slower for trans women. While we met our recruitment goals for lesbian and bisexual women, and exceeded the goals for gay, bisexual and other sexually diverse men, in three months we had only met half of our target for trans women. We then met with the trans peer researcher, who described the many participation barriers experienced by trans women, including time constraints due to precarious jobs including street-based sex work. Additionally, she shared how trans women in this context were a mobile group and precariously housed, and this created difficulties in making appointments for research interviews. We decided to be patient and increase the recruitment timeframe, and within six months we engaged our anticipated goal of 140 persons.

There was also rapid turnover in trans peer researchers during this study, as the first peer researcher was successful in an asylum claim to leave Jamaica. On another occasion, I arrived in Kingston to conduct some research training at JASL and the trans peer navigator did not show up. We were unable to reach her, and later found out that she had been arrested and jailed for simply walking around the prior evening doing outreach work. The specific barriers that trans women experience, including police harassment and arrest, required flexibility by and understanding from researchers. In 2019 and 2020, I was contacted by lawyers in the USA to provide expert witness testimonials for trans women seeking asylum from Jamaica. They used our published study findings to support successful claims, instilling in me a deep understanding of the ways by which research in rights-constrained contexts can be used in advocacy.

We found in our cross-sectional survey that a large proportion of LGBT persons were sex work involved and more likely to experience poorer sexual and mental health outcomes. The national sex work survey in Jamaica at that time only included cisgender women. We therefore focused the last part of the study on a survey to include sex working cisgender men, cisgender women, and trans women. Findings highlighted unmet HIV testing and care needs among sex working cisgender men and trans women and identified additional gender-specific HIV prevention and care needs. This reflects the potential for iterative approaches to research that follow up and explore health needs among marginalized groups with an intersectional lens. We first explored sex work and linkages to health outcomes among LGBT persons, and then among sex workers we explored gender and sexual orientation differences in health outcomes.

Taken together this research example emphasizes the importance of the relationship between the researchers and the researched. Centering the voices and experiences of the researched, in this case LGBT young persons in Jamaica, revealed dissonance between narratives that focus on the need for legal change and local knowledge of contextual realities that prioritize community-level change. Local LGBT celebrations were held in private spaces and prioritized, in this example, love and intimacy. Liberation can therefore be understood as fluid and changing—there will likely be a focus on advocacy and legal change in future Pride celebrations, and there have now been several public Pride celebrations. Changing research direction to align with and build on community needs and interests can cultivate research and service engagement. Doing so, also highlights the importance of praxis and dialogical knowledge, whereby research can help us learn how to better serve persons categorized as hard to reach.

2.2 In Conversation—Nicolette Richardson (Née Jones)

Carmen: *I want to talk about the concept with you of relationality, how we can be changed by our interactions with others. There was almost a reciprocal interaction where we tried to meet the needs that came up in our research. What things stands out for you from the research?*

Nicolette: *This is probably one of the most important pieces of work I have done in my life because it unveiled so much. We had been working with these populations (gay, bisexual and other men who have sex with men, trans women, lesbian and bisexual women) for a very long time. Why had we not spoken to them in this kind of way before?*

We are providing services, we are meeting their need for clinical health care. But we're not talking about their emotional health. You know, how are you even surviving? What do your finances look like? All of those things. It was very eye opening for me. What was also a really big thing was even in all these moments of despair, there was still so much hope, a sense of community and amazing stories.

I remember this one guy who identified as a man who had sex with men. He was speaking in our focus group about how his mother saw that he was interested in hairdressing and she bought him a mannequin to practice on. His father also bought him hairdressing supplies. This was so eye opening for me, because in most of the other focus groups we did, the theme was pretty much "I get beat up every day. This is the hardship I'm facing everyday". But this man's example was a glimmer of hope. Something that showed goodness in the midst of everything else. Goodness is hard to see, especially when our team's trans research assistants spent the night in jail because they were trying to do some outreach with trans women. They were jailed because police thought that was a good way to keep trans woman off the streets. So, in all of these stories, and all of these terrible things that were happening, that story really gave me a lot of hope and helped me going forward for the next two years of the project.

Carmen: *I remember that story. One thing I remember, and this is not the hopeful story you just mentioned, was when I asked about decriminalization of homosexuality and one of the gay men participants said we should not focus on that. That we needed to change the community attitudes first or there is going to be a huge backlash. I thought, wow, we actually assume that we know what's best—decriminalization. But actually, there is a lot of nuance there.*

Nicolette: *I think that also highlighted the importance of including the people you're advocating for in your advocacy efforts. Because, yes, it is good for us to work towards decriminalization, but what does it mean for the people who have to go through this process every day? It seems like a great thing to do. But what does it really mean for their daily lives?*

Carmen: *I remember the focus group with trans women there were many stories of experiencing violence.*

Nicolette: *Yeah, I feel that the majority of trans experiences at that time would have been pretty sad and pretty violent. There are a lot more good stories now* *coming out because of the work that we did, and because of the spotlight we put on trans women. Initially we felt that there were probably fifteen to twenty trans women. But we got over a hundred trans people to respond. We highlighted some key struggles that they experience—there are so many layers to the trans experience in Jamaica. There was a lot of confusion regarding identity, which is why research studies had subsumed trans women as gay and bisexual men.*

Carmen: *What do you think when people say that gay and bisexual men, trans women or lesbians in Jamaica are hard to reach?*

Nicolette: *There were times when we thought the same thing, but you have to think about other avenues, maybe even unconventional ones. If I am sitting in my office everyday typing up these documents about advocacy for all of these groups, I do not know how to reach out to them. I am not a part of the community and they are not going to want to speak to me even if I can find them. What you really have to do, I don't want to say 'go underground', but you really have to find those grassroots resources that connect with these communities. And I do not think that you should insert yourself in this space. Our method of finding key informants from the community, hiring and training them specifically to conduct this research project, was the best way to go. In some instances, I did support the research assistants. I did not feel as if we had enough trust within the community for me to go along with the trans research assistant. Instead, I listened to the recorded interviews and then gave her feedback. So sometimes you have to know when to step back. You have to trust your research assistants and trust that you trained them well.*

Carmen: *Why do you think that we were so successful getting over nine hundred and fifty LGBT persons to participate in this research study?*

Nicolette: *I think because it was a three-pronged approach. It was the individual interviews, then the focus group discussion, and then the surveys. People realized that it wasn't just "wham, bam, thank you, ma'am". We wanted to see you progressing through this. So not just, "You have given me this information. Goodbye. Thank you." No, we want to see you again. We are giving you this card to come to access services at our office. That continuum that we took the respondents on was different than other research projects they had done. Yes, we did include an honorarium and other research projects have done that. But I think the difference was that we wanted to see them again. It was not just "Thanks for the research. Bye. We will never see you again."*

When I went to meet with the respondents along with the research assistant, I spoke to them about the process. I let them know what we were going to do and what our anticipated outcomes were and informed them that if they wanted to help us in any other way, they should reach out to me. In this way they can see themselves in this research project. Not simply that they have collected money in exchange for data that they have no idea what you're using it for. We also had a pretty good connection with the team because we had chosen really good research assistants. As a side note, asking them to refer a friend was a great way to increase trust among participants.

Carmen: *I also felt we were patient, especially with the trans women. We waited six months to reach our goal for participants. Most people want to recruit all of their participants in a month or two.*

Nicolette: *That was also very helpful. The timeline of the project was flexible so we could iron some things out, because we had no idea if we could reach 140 trans women. Definitely not. Just being patient and building up that trust and those footholds in those communities. Even right now there is still that connection with these trans woman. This research project was a way of showing that we want to reach you, and we want to hear what you have to say. That is what creates this trusting relationship, which is really integral to working with vulnerable populations.*

Carmen: *Thank you. I want to ask for your feedback on something. When I look back on this study, I thought how responsive the community partner we worked with was to take the qualitative findings and apply for a grant to do more trans specific services. For me that really felt as if they were demonstrating their care about trans women and tried to meet the needs of the community.*

Nicolette: *Working very intimately with the qualitative data, it was really very interesting to see all of the different connections that we could make. I remember sharing the new findings with my office mate at the time. And then in staff meetings we would say, well, how can we reach trans people? We have all of this funding for men who have sex with men, but what about this whole population of people that we are not reaching because of the restrictions from funding agencies? So, the Elton John Foundation grant came up and we used our findings to make the case that we needed to provide services for trans women. I also think that this demonstrates progressive leadership. We also started to include trans women's issues and needs in our capacity-building workshops with health care providers, and in our conversations with other LGBT agencies in Jamaica.*

So, we did not just sit down and look at this amazing data and say, well, we did this. We actually were and still are acting. My colleagues are still actively working with trans populations in different ways to ensure that they are being reached with these specific services. There was also sensitization training with the police we were doing through another violence against women campaign, and we found opportunities to insert our findings with trans women.

Carmen: *That is so inspiring. What I also really appreciated was the respectful way the agency acknowledged and addressed knowledge gaps. They hired one of the trans community agencies to do a trans sensitivity training for the staff at each site.*

Nicolette: *In our work we are sensitized to the different issues surrounding sex workers and men who have sex with men, but not to trans issues. It was powerful to hear about trans experiences. Two people, a trans woman and a trans man, came to speak to each of the three chapters in the agency. We opened the floor for them to share their experiences because, while we know scientific things and have other kinds of knowledge and are generally sensitized, we needed to hear their experiences and how they are having to traverse life. For instance, they shared how they were "sneaking around" to access certain clinical services like access to hormones. How healthcare providers refuse to call them by their name and preferred gender. You* *would not have known these experiences if you did not go to that training or had not spoken to this person. We also were able to see the differences in realities for trans women as opposed to trans men. It broadened our horizons and how we can extend our services to reach these specific groups.*

Carmen: *What do you think about this idea that me, you and the whole research team of peer navigators were learning from the participants. For me, I felt like I learned a lot. How marginalized people were, but also how there was a lot of bravery and community organizing. It was very humbling for me.*

Nicolette: *It was a great experience and we had regular meetings with all members of our research team to provide support if they needed to talk about anything. They were invited to schedule meetings with the counsellor or the therapist, because they were exposed to some very heavy stories about the realities of people's lives. It is difficult not to internalize those things or to become consumed with all the negative stories that you're being told while you are trying to remain neutral in your research assistant capacity. A few people talked to me and said they needed to take a break to offload. There are people who had been doing this work for years before and said they had never connected with people in this kind of way. When hearing these stories, it is heartbreaking, but it also made us more motivated to work to create a better, safer space for us all to co-exist.*

I felt with all this information we were collecting, we had to do something about the current situation. I was heartened to see the trans advocacy groups were growing and expanding into more rural communities. In all of this despair, we were creating community and in lots of different ways working to advocate for a better quality of life. I am sure they are still using this research today because of how poignant it was, because of the relevance to the whole situation of men who have sex with men, women who have sex with women, and trans men and women in Jamaica.

Carmen: *I think that is amazing that there was actually the thought and the action that we need to also take care of the research assistants who were holding these stories. It was still tough to get the lesbian and bisexual woman. I remember I came the focus group and nobody showed up.*

Nicolette: *Yes, it is a more guarded thing for lesbian women. It goes back to trust. They do not see why you are talking to them about HIV or AIDS, they do not see the connection. Why should I talk to you? What is the point? In framing the messages through the research, I focused on stepping back to let them know that this was not just about HIV, it was to talk about how you are accessing services and to understand what we can do to improve their quality of life overall.*

We reinforced the point that we are not trying to give them an HIV test, what we are trying to do is simply have a conversation. Then a few showed up. It was very difficult for those who identified at the time as butch lesbians because they are very susceptible to verbal and physical attacks. It is more difficult for people to understand why you are dressing this way and behaving this way. They get more persecution. So, they were a bit more guarded to speak about their experiences. I remember one girl saying that she was a butch, and when she became pregnant, everybody was surprised that she could have wanted a child. Then there were so many other stories of butch lesbians who were raped. People were thinking that if she was raped, then she would turn away from being a lesbian—this whole idea of 'corrective' rape. How would that affect her and continue to affect her? There were other stories from feminine presenting lesbians, and how they sometimes escaped those harsh persecutions, but cannot be open to their families or show any kind of PDA (public display of affection). That specific focus group was a very interesting dynamic hearing from the different groups of lesbians and how their persecution or levels of discrimination varied based on their gender presentation.

Carmen: *What do you think about the idea of community care within the LGBT spectrum?*

Nicolette: *I think it does exist. It is the only way people can really survive and thrive. I remember the very first focus group discussion with trans women in New Kingston and everybody was there talking about survival, and what that looks like on the street. They created tiny communities. They were able to bounce ideas off of each other and support one another. Now, the other side of this is that it is very easy to become clique-ish. You may know those people over there, but you and your girls have been through a lot and you are not going to let anyone else in, and that can cause friction. Yes, there is a community of care, but because of all the obstacles that exist for trans women, men who have sex with men, and lesbians, these communities of care can also reinforce societal pressures. There are hierarchies that exist within the communities too that may be based on society's norms.*

Carmen: *There was almost some sort of self-regulation. I will never forget that time that one person in the group was from a low-income community. He was saying "I am fine if I do not bring anybody home. Nobody is going to harm me because I have a community". I was shocked. I saw a very feminine presenting man from a low-income neighbourhood who felt protected by his community.*

Nicolette: *That is part of the acceptance or tolerance of being gay and acting feminine. What Jamaicans generally do not want to think about is the fact that you are actually attracted to another men. So, yes, you are in this community, yes, you are one of us. But if you bring somebody else home, then that is a whole different thing.*

Carmen: *It is sort of a 'don't ask, don't tell' situation. What is interesting to me, and I do not know if you have this experience, but I feel like I am always defending Jamaica. The reaction when I share that I do LGBT research in Jamaica is an automatic response that "Oh, my God, it is so terrible, they are so homophobic". I feel that while there is stigma and homophobia, there is actually, like the example you gave, a mom and dad supporting their gay son to become a hairdresser. There is the trans woman whose sister still supports her. There are all of these people mobilizing. There is so much nuance and complexity, buried under this stereotype.*

Nicolette: *I think that is what this project showed me. Yes, some terrible things happen. Yes, it can be terribly violent, but we are moving away from that. It is difficult to change people's minds. There is a gradual progression. It used to be physical and sexual violence. Now it is more verbal, people will say whatever they want to say to you on the street. Yes, that is still not okay, but it is progress. We are moving to a place of indifference. People might think that that is not growth or something to celebrate, but it is if we can prevent more gay men, more lesbian* *women, more trans men and trans women from being hurt. That is really the whole point. They will have to deal with verbal backlash, it is not going to be great for their self-esteem overall or for their journey to becoming their true selves. But we are keeping them safe generally and through programs and initiatives, we are providing the space for them to be able to talk about and hopefully overcome these psychological obstacles. While moving to a place of indifference is not the best strategy, I would say it has been a win for us in this instance. Even though we have spoken about physical abuse and 'corrective' rape, that has generally been a thing of the past because of these communities that they have been able to create.*

People on the LGBTQ spectrum are leaving home sooner, and they are able to create these close-knit families that will basically protect them. I remember one of the peer coordinators took care of a few trans people in her community. She would bring three or four girls to stay with her and they would figure out how they were going to make money. If they had any issues, they would talk to her. It was a way for them to move beyond this one survival option: sex work. She started selling clothes and she would employ some of the girls. That was a pretty massive thing.

Carmen: *Another thing I learned was the importance of recognizing my own biases and cultural expectations. I remember in a focus group where one of the guys said there was going to be a Pride march and then a hardware store sold out of machetes as people were planning to stand alongside the road and attack the parade. In some of the in-depth interviews people were saying, "this is Jamaica, we do not need to walk down the street holding our partner's hand—we just want to walk down the street beside them". There was this idea that maybe liberation is going to look different in Jamaica. Maybe it doesn't need to look like New York.*

Nicolette: *That is the value of speaking to the group. Because in our eyes we believe you should be able to do this. Why shouldn't you be able to walk down the street holding your partner's hand? Well, the group was thinking that we need to work up to that. Let us not start there. Let us just say we want to be able to get a job and keep a job. Let us just start at the beginning. So many lessons in those groups came because we are trying to see the bigger picture and way down the line, but they were saying, "we have to crawl before we can walk. So, what are some small steps you could be taking?"*

We needed to take those small steps to address issues they were having. So, we started having workshops with gay and bisexual men, using topics that came up from the focus group discussions to fuel those workshops. I remember one of the people from the focus group said, "why can't we ever talk about romance and sex and relationships? Why does everybody focus on HIV?" We then did a whole series about relationships and what you're looking for in relationships and how that relates to personal growth. Those seemingly small things were able to change our conversation with gay men, even the ones who were already accessing our services. Our services are very heavily HIV and STI focused. Aside from all the talk about protection and getting tested, they are regular people who are having regular issues, who do not want to talk about HIV all the time. This project also helped us to change our messaging. Back in the day the communication was pretty much just "Get tested, get tested. Getting tested is a thing you need to do." But we learned to soften the message and make it more palatable, more likeable, more relatable, more sexy. We are crafting messages that people can really connect with.

We were carving out these spaces where we can really do something for the population we're working with, this meant focusing on just being able to connect and being able to have some social relationships. It is about being free and getting out there, as well as supporting you if you want to get tested. I was learning and relearning how to really connect with our clients. Yes, healthcare services are great, but social services are also important. So, offering counselling services free of charge as well as hosting social events are very important. This is how we get into those spaces, where people will be able to trust us as allies, advocates and service providers. How can we be seen as an ally?

Carmen: *What would you like to say for the next researcher who wants to work in places, for example, where it is illegal to be gay? Or places where people strategically choose to be more underground?*

Nicolette: *You have to be open to learning and to modifying your plan. We modified plans so many times based on the new information we were able to find. The reality is people need to be flexible, to know that these are people—not lab rats. These are people with lives and complex things going on. You cannot just expect that they are going to show up every day for your survey. They are people first, and that perspective needs to be at the front of your research. It is finding the right people to connect with and knowing that you do not have to insert yourself in every single interaction.*

Listen, wait, and really meet people where they are. We realized, working with trans women that we needed to pay for transportation for research assistants to meet these participants where they were. For the focus group, we provided transportation to the meeting place. Researchers need to be aware of those things and adjust their research, and their funding if possible, to develop different ways to reach the population. It is not a one size fits all approach. These are the other pieces of the puzzle that may not be visible from the surface.

2.3 Applying Concepts of Context and Storytelling to Understand the Hard to Reach

Our interactions and relations with others have the potential to lead to fresh perspectives and ways of living. *Relationality* also encompasses connections with diverse persons and places: "a relational account of space argues that responsibilities arise not only through direct actions and implications, but also through simply being part of wider systems of injustice and inequality elsewhere" (Darling, 2009, p. 1946). Interactions with others are shaped by larger power structures, however, and relationships can play a role in maintaining or disrupting inequitable power dynamics. Relational perspectives consider how these interactions can be used to develop and transform power through building equitable connections and alliances with people and organizations. Communities of responsibility can include persons in close proximity, humanitarian crises, and persons who are marginalized from ongoing effects of historical events and actions, including slavery and colonization (Darling, 2009). Relationality includes both expressive dimensions, such as providing the opportunity to work on priorities identified as important with collaborating persons and organizations, as well as instrumental dimensions that include sharing skills, resources and motivation to enact social change. Relational transactions and processes are central to shaping identities, nurturing wellbeing, building communities, and producing and sharing knowledge. Context and storytelling enhance understanding of relationality and were central to our success in connecting with participants in this research example of working with LGBT youth in Jamaica.

2.4 Context

> Shifting the unit of analysis and agent of change from individuals, and individual risk behaviour, to environments, shifts how we think about responsibility for harm—from constituting individuals alone as responsible for their behaviour to tackling the socio-political situations and structures in which individuals find themselves (Rhodes, 2002, p. 88).

Stigma and discrimination are socially organized and shaped by history (for instance, slavery and colonization), geography (including rural, urban settings), political environment (laws, policies), culture (values, beliefs, religion), and gender norms (including roles and expectations) (Harnois, Bastos, Campbell, & Keith, 2019). Social, material, and political contexts result in stigma being differentially experienced and negotiated within and between contexts. This means that in countries such as Jamaica, where the criminalization of same sex practices was introduced under British Colonial rule, and persons of African descent were forcibly brought to Jamaica to work as slaves, that these colonial histories have a role in shaping current day manifestations of stigma. Stereotypes of Jamaica as a homophobic country largely persist without a concurrent analysis of the ongoing impact of these histories of colonization, slavery, and British homophobic rule (Stewart, 2017).

Semugoma et al. have discussed three ironies of African homophobia that are salient to understanding homophobia in Jamaica and other formerly colonized countries (Semugoma, Nemande, & Baral, 2012). First, the majority of laws globally criminalizing same-sex practices were introduced by colonial rulers, who have since abolished these laws within their own countries and labelled them discriminatory. This is true in Jamaica, where the current laws criminalizing same sex practices under the 'Offences Against the Person Act', 1864 were introduced under British colonial rule. (Ramon Mendos, 2019) The UK's 'Offences Against the Person Act' was repealed in 1967 in England and Wales, in 1981 in Scotland, and 1982 in Northern Ireland (Ramon Mendos, 2019).

The second irony is that in Sub-Saharan Africa as well as in Jamaican media and discourse, LGBT rights movements are often characterized as Western imports.

However, it is also true that Western actors have supported anti-LGBT movements in the Global South, such as USA evangelical Christian movements in Uganda. The USA has a long history, enforced through the US President's Emergency Plan for AIDS Relief (PEPFAR) until 2004, of supporting faith-based organizations opposed to LGBT rights to implement HIV programming. As a result, Semugoma et al. describe how "Africa has become a battleground for developed countries' so-called cultural wars" (Semugoma et al., 2012, p. 312). Jamaica, alongside other countries, is a PEPFAR recipient, receiving more than four million US dollars between 2010 and 2018 support to the National HIV/STI program (USAID, 2010). Yet the Mexico City Policy 'global gag rule' is a US federal policy reimplemented in 2017 that bars global health foreign funding to any agency that provides information, services or advocacy related to abortion (amfAR, 2019). This limits funding to the program's implementing partners across the Global South who provide access to comprehensive sexual and reproductive health services. Service disruptions arising from the gag rule particularly impact key populations in the HIV responses, including LGBT persons, as the agencies that offer affirmative, respectful HIV prevention and testing services for LGBT persons are also more likely to be the places that offer comprehensive sexual and reproductive health information (amfAR, 2019; Mavodza, Goldman, & Cooper, 2019). This example shows tensions between HIV funding that has the potential to be health promoting, and US policies that harm LGBT persons by disrupting and reducing access to health services (Alliance for Health Policy and Systems Research, 2012; amfAR, 2019; Mavodza et al., 2019; Singh & Karim, 2017). Additionally, framing LGBT liberation as a Western agenda overlooks local LGBT histories in Sub-Saharan Africa, the Caribbean, and other contexts (Dlamini, 2006; Epprecht, 2009; Ramsay, 2009).

The third irony is that when there is no documentation of the lives and stories of LGBT persons—including their HIV vulnerabilities—in rights-constrained contexts such as Jamaica then LGBT communities can be overlooked in HIV research, programming, and funding opportunities. Our team experienced this when some local agencies questioned how we were able to reach so many trans women since they were unaware of their existence. Taken together, these ironies signal the need to carefully examine historical and current impacts of colonization on persons labelled hard to reach. Rather than largely framing homophobia as endemic to 'local cultures' it can be viewed as a legacy of colonialism.

2.4.1 Conceptualizing Context

There are myriad approaches to conceptualizing context. Context, for instance, has symbolic, material, and relational dimensions (Campbell et al., 2013; Campbell & Cornish, 2012). Symbolic context refers to the socio-cultural meanings, values, and beliefs that shape understandings of self and others. These can include stigma and gender inequitable norms that shape who is (and is not) recognized as worthy and deserving of dignity and rights. Material context includes resources and experiences. Such resources include access to food, housing, employment and economic security that contribute to not only survival but also recognition of value and worth. Material contexts include being able to use one's skills and to practise agency (Campbell & Cornish, 2012). In this chapter's example, we could see that JASL offered support groups that were immediately needed to support trans women, while continuing advocacy work for LGBT rights. JASL also provided employment skills training tailored to trans women's interests, including hairdressing. Relational contexts include recognition of rights, participation of marginalized communities, healthcare treatment, social support and social capital. This social capital can be bonding (e.g. building relationships within the LGBT community) as well as bridging, whereby persons who experience marginalization can build relationships with persons holding socio-economic and political power in order to advance their goals (Bourdieu, 1986; Nhamo, Campbell, & Gregson, 2010; Putnam, 2001). Participating in formal (e.g. organizational HIV support group, church group) and informal (e.g. family, neighbourhood) community groups and social networks can spark dialogue that contests inequitable social norms, result in a sharing of lived experiences that fosters empathy, and can build solidarity to effect positive social change (Campbell et al., 2013).

These Indigenous social relations can foster what is referred to as HIV-competent communities (Nhamo et al., 2010), in which persons share HIV knowledge and strategies to overcome barriers to engaging in HIV prevention and identify strengths and protective factors. However there remain challenges if misinformation is spread in social networks or inequitable norms are reinforced and upheld. Enabling environments are health promoting—they foster solidarity, resilience, resistance, and belonging through amplifying voices of, and access to power among, marginalized persons (Campbell & Cornish, 2012; Rhodes, 2009). Contexts therefore co-produce both risks and protective factors in structures, interactions, and daily practices.

Rhodes has described some of the social and physical environmental spaces and mechanisms that produce risks and responses (Rhodes, 2002, 2009). Contextual factors include policies, responses, and programs. Examining the micro-social environment can shed insight into what might constitute a "recipe for an epidemic" (Rhodes, 2002, p. 87). The risk environment includes social, physical, economic and policy spaces and situations at micro and macro levels that increase or reduce harm (Rhodes, 2002, 2009). Micro-level risk environments include perceived health risks and practices, community norms, rules and values, social relationships and networks, and neighbourhood contexts (Rhodes, 2002). These are different from, but shaped by, the macro-level risk environments that comprise social, economic, racial and gender inequities, laws and policies. Physical environments include exposure to other health issues (such as geographic spaces where there may be high prevalence of HIV), and geographically prescribed migration and tourist routes and other spaces that may have a high population density and social disparities (e.g. prisons) (Rhodes, 2002, p. 90).

Social factors, individual health practices, and the physical environment converge and interact in ways that can amplify or decrease exposure to harmful social and health outcomes (Rhodes, 1997). In this way, "the physical environment may ...

help create and sustain the micro social relations of risk" (Rhodes, 1997, p. 90). There are also contextually specific social meanings behind 'risk' practices—changing the social context is therefore vital to reducing risk factors (Rhodes, 1997, 2009). Framing social relationships as the unit of analysis, rather than individual decision making, centres power im/balances within social systems and interactions as key elements that shape risk decision making ('risk rationalities') (Rhodes, 2009). Rather than being discrete categories, micro and macro levels overlap and interact in many ways, as do social, physical, policy and economic dimensions of the environment. For instance, in Jamaica, the macro policy decision of LGBT criminalization sanctions healthcare discrimination that influences LGBT persons' knowledge of and access to HIV preventive resources, in turn shaping micro level practices regarding decision making regarding HIV testing and care in stigmatizing environments. This environmental analysis demonstrates how risk is socially situated (Rhodes, 1997, 2002, 2009).

Beyond this, Rhodes delineates the mechanisms by which environments can influence risk. These include *susceptibility*, the likelihood one will be influenced or harmed, as well as *vulnerability*, socio-economic environmental features that influence the odds of experiencing a disproportionate morbidity and mortality of a particular illness (Barnett, Whiteside, Khodakevich, Kruglov, & Steshenko, 2000). For instance, the odds of HIV infection reflect susceptibility, influenced by macro-level factors such as background rates of HIV and other STIs, and micro-level factors such as consistent condom use. HIV vulnerability, on the other hand, reflects the ability to respond to and mitigate the effects of HIV, and is shaped by macro-level factors such as poverty and the criminalization of same sex practices, and at the micro-level, factors such as access to condoms and lubricant, and the ability to access non-stigmatizing HIV testing. In Jamaica, susceptibility includes the high background HIV and STI prevalence among gay, bisexual and other MSM, and vulnerability includes the ways that LGBT stigma and criminalization constrain access to HIV prevention information, resources (such as condoms), and testing and care services.

2.4.2 How Our Work Was Able to Address Context

Ultimately, in our work in Jamaica, we aimed to build capacity and skills among LGBT persons who were hired and trained as peer researchers across all study phases. Providing payment as well as training produced material contexts that valued peer researchers' work and built confidence in communication and research skills. We also aimed to increase knowledge and health engagement among LGBT participants by increasing access to and uptake of HIV and syphilis testing and JASL's outreach services. Peer navigators were closely involved in working with community stakeholders to facilitate recruitment. One unintended social consequence of this was that the qualitative findings could be used rapidly by the community partner to apply for and receive external funding to create support groups with trans women (bonding capital). The trans affirmative service delivery training across JASL sites increased the ability of staff working to build strong, respectful relationships with trans clients. This reflects bridging social capital. It also showed how it is not always information provision that is required to prevent HIV, it is also the chance to discuss and process this information for integration into real life (Nhamo et al., 2010).

Throughout the study, we tried to understand the range of experiences of stigma (symbolic context) among LGBT persons, and to use this knowledge to develop alternative, less stigmatizing approaches to HIV information and testing. For instance, HIV-related and LGBT stigma converge to reduce access to information and uptake of HIV prevention and testing resources. By focusing on the continued engagement of LGBT persons across study phases, and hiring LGBT persons to conduct outreach to engage and link participants with HIV and syphilis testing and information, we started to break down access barriers to HIV resources. Stigmatizing contexts, and high HIV prevalence, among gay men and transgender women in Jamaica, held symbolic value for the project both in Jamaica and internationally when we published and presented our findings. On the day we planned a community forum to share the study findings, and invited speakers with lived experiences of sex work and LGBT stigma, a rainstorm struck. The streets were completely flooded. I was so disappointed. But colleagues assured me that people would come—they would simply arrive late. This was true, and more than one hundred and fifty persons, including LGBT persons, sex workers, government and non-government agencies, arrived despite the heavy rain. We hired a local youth dance troupe who created dances and songs regarding ending LGBT and HIV stigma. These felt like small yet important wins in improving the symbolic context—people came to learn about the study findings and services for LGBT persons in Jamaica improved. Not only did community collaborator staff improve their ability to provide trans affirmative care, but most LGBT study participants opted to receive an HIV and/or syphilis test and in turn accessed care and support.

The relational context likely played the biggest role in helping the research team to engage with LGBT youth in Jamaica. We attempted to facilitate the meaningful participation of LGBT persons by hiring a team of peer navigators. They built bonding social capital with other LGBT persons, offering support and understanding of local experiences, and verifying safe spaces for study activities and HIV and syphilis testing. This approach helped the study nearly double the anticipated participant sample size. By quickly identifying gaps in trans knowledge and competency, and engaging a local trans group to deliver training, JASL built bridging capital with trans communities. The confidence and trust the peer navigators exhibited in JASL to identify these knowledge gaps also suggest the importance of building spaces for transformative communication in the research setting.

2.4.3 How Our Work Was Unable to Address Context

The material context is difficult to transform. Although we provided salaries to peer navigators, we were unable to effect larger changes for LGBT youth in Jamaica. Poverty, including a lack of employment and housing opportunities due to stigma and discrimination, is a structural driver of HIV vulnerability that extended beyond the study's reach. Despite our findings that demonstrated multi-level contexts of HIV vulnerabilities, it took 3 years and four grant applications before we received additional funding to build on initial work undertaken. The funding we did receive was only one-fifth of what we had applied for. This resulted in our not being able to fully harness the capacity of the peer navigators, and we lost the momentum and connections with many smaller collaborating agencies.

Conversations with colleagues about funding challenges revealed that Jamaica's classification as a middle-income country rendered it a low priority context for funders. It could be the relatively small (~150) number of trans persons we anticipated that we could include in future studies. As a research project funded to focus on HIV, we were not able to expand to address the other environmental factors that profoundly impacted health and wellbeing among LGBT persons such as housing. The case study presented here reflected our flexible approach to respond to young LGBT persons' needs, understand the micro and macro contexts of their lives, and to keep continued engagement over a 3-year study. Through applying this approach, we realized that LGBT youth in this rights-constrained context were not in fact so very hard to reach.

2.5 Storytelling

> Common humanity expressed through stories connects story-tellers and audiences, clinicians and patients . . . the corollary to the danger of stories is that stories make people less scared. Fear comes from uncertainty, misunderstanding, and a failure to recognize humanity in one another (Harman, 2020, p. 777).

Stories can enhance understanding of lived experiences, meanings, identities, complexity and politics embedded in everyday ways knowing and being (Harman, 2016; Lewis, 2011). Stories offer new perspectives that can disrupt preconceptions and conventional, master narratives rooted in privilege (e.g. racial, sexual orientation, class) to expose social injustices (Denzin, 2008; Solórzano & Yosso, 2002). In turn, these fresh ways of seeing and thinking can open new possibilities for how we act. Stories include both internal (the content) and external (the process) narratives (Banks, 2001). These narratives can provide space for voices to be heard that may often be elided or disregarded (Harman, 2020; Solórzano & Yosso, 2002). Stories of persons who are marginalized can be considered *counter-stories* that uncover and challenge dominant narratives; they also reflect resistance and socio-cultural and political survival (Solórzano & Yosso, 2002). Storytelling can connect with the reader emotionally and cognitively. This emotional connection can foster empathy by helping us to see ourselves in others and, in turn, this can serve as a reminder, as described in the opening quotation, of our common humanity. Gathering and amplifying stories from persons constructed as hard to reach can provide HIV researchers with insight into barriers to research participation and can help us identify and challenge inaccurate preconceptions.

Feminist perspectives honor everyday lived experiences as valuable sources of knowledge (Harman, 2018; Weldon, 2006). Stories from communities help us understand how HIV is viewed and experienced and what might be appropriate interventions (and for who). Stories can also reflect experiential knowledge that may run counter to scientific knowledge and government policy (Harman, 2020). For instance, the conversation with Nicolette earlier in this chapter explored participants' view that we need to focus on changing hearts and minds before changing laws. Experiential knowledge revealed that decriminalization alone will not stop—and may in fact exacerbate—stigma, discrimination and hate crimes targeting LGBT persons in Jamaica. These stories point to locally grounded solutions to stigma—in this case, the complex but important work of changing community norms. This contextual focus expands beyond a focus on global decriminalization (Johnson, 2019; Ramon Mendos, 2019). Participant narratives also highlighted sexual and physical violence by police targeting LGBT persons. Providing a platform for storytelling in rights-constrained contexts can directly benefit persons' lives. I have served as an expert witness for LGBT persons from Jamaica seeking asylum in other countries on multiple occasions: our documentation of police violence was key to success in these cases, providing an example of the way in which stories can be told and harnessed as spaces for resistance (Lewis, 2011).

There are dangers, however, in storytelling regarding whose stories are told, how stories are used, and who has access to the accounts. There is a challenge to balance oppression and agency; and because stories often follow an individual character as a protagonist, it may be harder to reflect heterogeneity of experiences as well as structural inequities. This can result in stories focused on individual suffering and hardship. As Harman (2020, p. 777) has put it: "Too often stories are used in ways that allow audiences to eat the trauma of the story-teller ... this presents a conundrum to story-telling in global health: how to communicate humanity in a way that does not feast on the trauma of others". Conversely, stories can fall into the *instrumentalist trap* and portray persons who are marginalized as overly resilient in overcoming structural inequities (Harman, 2016). These tropes of a victim or hero underscore the need for stories that reflect the tension between structural violence and agency among LGBT persons in Jamaica, and the diverse and dynamic stories among LGBT persons.

Stories can also reveal how larger socio-economic, political and global structures constrain agency. As researchers we can notice and question the framing of non-Western cultures as essentially homophobic and dangerous places for LGBT persons, and LGBT persons in these places as invisible and passive. Such portrayals position Western contexts as progressive places populated by human rights guardians (Logie & Gibson, 2013). Research ethics boards in Western contexts such as

Canada often construct LGBT persons as highly vulnerable in research, which in turn may make it challenging and time consuming to obtain research ethics approval. This can be a deterrent to conducting research in contexts that may benefit from a better understanding of LGBT peoples' lives (Tufford, Newman, Brennan, Craig, & Woodford, 2012).

Understanding storytelling as research/research as storytelling can also help researchers to consider power asymmetries between themselves and research participants. In particular, we can harness the power of stories in research to illuminate the ways that people balance agency within contextual constraints and how they negotiate fluid dynamics of vulnerability. Our research project in Jamaica for example, intentionally balanced a focus on structural violence (stigma, criminalization, violence targeting LGBT persons) with a concern for LGBT agency (supportive relations, resistance, community building). To avoid producing harm by propagating a single narrative, we asked about stigma and acceptance, coping strategies, lessons learned, and advice participants wished to share with other LGBT persons. Research can leverage stories as a tool to disrupt representations of people and places by raising awareness of participants' internal narratives (lived experiences, hopes, dreams) and the researcher's external narrative (designing and conducting research). In this way, research holds the potential to create space and audience for the voices of marginalized persons to be heard on a global platform.

Counter-stories can also foster community among persons at the margins, question the knowledge of persons with power (e.g. researcher), and reveal hidden possibilities and realities (Solórzano & Yosso, 2002). Counter-stories invite us to reflect on our own internal/external narratives and when they are challenged by the stories we hear. For instance, I had first to be aware of my own ideas of what queer liberation can/should look like and my love of Pride celebrations, in order to understand my initial reaction of disappointment when listening to stories that diverged from these ideas. Recognizing the stories being told about a particular place, person or group, and about HIV itself, can help us to disengage from and start to unravel these stories. People—and contexts—are dynamic, and in turn stories adapt and change (Harman, 2020). Stories are shaped in larger material, relational and symbolic contexts. How then can we engage with the heterogenous stories of people who are labelled hard to reach, and collaboratively share these stories to enhance understanding, empathy, solidarity and other possibilities?

2.6 Rethinking Hard to Reach Through a Focus on Context and Storytelling

The convergence of context and storytelling discussed in this chapter can best be understood through the concept of place. *Place* can be considered as geographical (e.g. a location's latitude, elevation) but also as phenomenological, reflecting the ways in which a place shapes physical, social and economic processes and social practices in a location (Agnew, 2011; Akesson, Burns, & Hordyk, 2017). Phenomenological approaches to place focus on interactions over the life course and within the environment, rather than individual level factors. This reinforces how "we always look at 'the world from somewhere, from a place ... knowledge is always and everywhere geographically contextual and reflexive" (Agnew, 2011, p. 21). Places are active and relational, shaping and being shaped by networks and interactions at the "convergence of different trajectories and histories" (Darling, 2009, p. 1938). Relational perspectives on place encourage *outwardlookingness* whereby we bring to light perspectives from insiders—as research participants—looking out (Darling, 2009). Other approaches to place emphasize the need to better understand the quality of place: what and who are there, and how people are interacting (Florida, 2003). Relational approaches to place require researchers to focus on heterogeneity within a particular place and its stories, and connections between a place and outside systems and places (Darling, 2009, 2010).

In research it is important to consider how our social practices produce our experience of a place—we are part of constructing the spatial other, including persons categorized as hard to reach. Places are fluid and dynamic, they have permeable boundaries, and they are comprised of diverse experiences (Agnew, 2011; Darling, 2010; Jones, 2009). Solidarity and resistance are connected to a shared sense of place (Agnew, 2011), yet the global stretching of socio-spatial relations can create a wider collective identity, solidarity, and sense of imagined community that extend a sense of responsibility beyond one place (Darling, 2009; Jones, 2009; Smith, 2016). The relational responsibilities discussed in this chapter include LGBT persons from places with more resources and rights (such as myself, a queer researcher from Canada) forming partnerships with LGBT persons from places with less resources and constrained rights (LGBT colleagues and allies in Jamaica). This collaboration was motivated from solidarity between LGBT persons as well as by the histories of colonization that contribute to current day constrained LGBT rights. Relational responsibilities can also extend beyond persons with shared social identities to address processes of caring for the 'other' (Smith, 2016) to view all lives as worthy of dignity and socio-economic inclusion: "relational spatial politics, of connected and constitutive responsibilities, seeks to challenge the ways in which others may be cast aside" (Darling, 2009, p. 1944). Research can therefore serve as a conduit to connect people within and between places for collective action.

Creating and sharing knowledge happens in the conversations between persons in different social and spatial contexts (Rutten, 2016). Social dynamics shape interactions that can stimulate or dampen knowledge sharing and creation. Relational approaches consider the opportunities for connection present in each place (Jones, 2009; Rutten, 2016). Research can therefore be the middle ground that connects the local, situated, underground knowledge of the hard to reach with the institutional knowledge of academia and social and health practitioners. It requires effort to bridge distances and connect with particular places and people, and our personal preferences and bonds with others inspire us to do so (Darling, 2009; Rutten, 2016). Distance can reduce our feelings of ethical obligation—widening our indifference to *others* (Darling, 2009; Smith, 2016). Our project in Jamaica included "multi-local anchored conversations" (Rutten, 2016, p. 172), whereby researchers from multiple countries (Canada, Jamaica) were involved in understanding locally situated knowledge and sharing findings with local and global audiences. The conceptualization of place as a trajectory, a meeting point, and as heterogeneous, reflects the contrasting experiences of marginalization and agency that LGBT youth shared with us as participants in this study.

Researchers working with persons labelled hard to reach should therefore be alert to multiple contextual dimensions, listen for what stories are told and untold, and notice how the places researchers occupy converge and diverge from the places in which persons labelled hard to reach dwell. Embracing a relational perspective can challenge the notion of place as inaccessible, or as having prescribed or proscribed boundaries, reflected in the term itself—hard to reach. Distancing ourselves from hard to reach places and people produces misunderstandings, knowledge gaps, and ultimately a lower feeling of responsibility for the 'other' (Rutten, 2016; Smith, 2016). As researchers wanting to connect with persons who may be considered hard to reach, we should consider the ways in which our power and relational responsibility "extend the spatial scope of our actions to those who are distant . . . responsibility does not simply proceed 'outwards', but implies a relationship between placed connections, territories and flows which is constantly shifting and constantly demanding" (Darling, 2009, p. 1945).

Building social environments that facilitate justice, HIV prevention and care engagement, and social and personal wellbeing, requires an understanding the multi-faceted nature of context and how our research may (and may not) influence this setting (Smith, 2016). Caring practices across spaces, or *caring-scapes*, include being responsive, attentive, and responsible toward distal and proximal others (Barnett & Land, 2007). By shifting the focus to the larger risk environment we can move away from labelling individuals as hard to reach and instead consider the risk context as a problematic barrier that needs to be dismantled (Rhodes, 1997, 2002, 2009). *Geographies of generosity* are perspectives that consider generosity as an expression of power that is integral to how we live together across time and space (Barnett & Land, 2007). As researchers we can harness this power and responsibility to build just, responsive, attentive and generous caring practices in research—to produce and mobilize knowledge and transform systems that create harm for people and places labelled hard to reach.

References

Agnew, J. (2011). Space and place. In J. A. Agnew & D. N. Livingstone (Eds.), *The SAGE handbook of geographical knowledge* (pp. 316–330). London: Sage.

Akesson, B., Burns, V., & Hordyk, S.-R. (2017). The place of place in social work: Rethinking the person-in-environment model in social work education and practice. *Journal of Social Work Education, 53*(3), 372–383.

Alliance for Health Policy and Systems Research. (2012). *Health policy and systems research: A methodology reader*. Geneva: World Health Organization.

amfAR. (2019). *The effect of the expanded Mexico city policy on HIV/AIDS programming: Evidence from the PEPFAR implementing partners survey*. amfAR: The Foundation for AIDS Research, New York.

Banks, M. (2001). *Visual methods in social research*. London: Sage.

Barnett, C., & Land, D. (2007). Geographies of generosity: Beyond the 'moral turn'. *Geoforum, 38*(6), 1065–1075.

Barnett, T., Whiteside, A., Khodakevich, L., Kruglov, Y., & Steshenko, V. (2000). The HIV/AIDS epidemic in Ukraine: Its potential social and economic impact. *Social Science and Medicine (1982), 51*(9), 1387–1403.

Bourdieu, P. (1986). The forms of capital. In J. G. Richardson (Ed.), *Handbook of theory and research for the sociology of education* (pp. 241–258). Westport, CT: Greenwood Press.

Campbell, C., & Cornish, F. (2012). How can community health programmes build enabling environments for transformative communication? Experiences from India and South Africa. *AIDS and Behavior, 16*(4), 847–857.

Campbell, C., Scott, K., Nhamo, M., Nyamukapa, C., Madanhire, C., Skovdal, M., Sherr, L., & Gregson, S. (2013). Social capital and HIV competent communities: The role of community groups in managing HIV/AIDS in rural Zimbabwe. *AIDS Care, 25*(suppl 1), S114–S122.

Darling, J. (2009). Thinking beyond place: The responsibilities of a relational spatial politics. *Geography Compass, 3*(5), 1938–1954.

Darling, J. (2010). Teaching and learning guide for: Thinking beyond place: The responsibilities of a relational spatial politics: Geography compass teaching and learning guide. *Geography Compass, 4*(6), 676–681.

Denzin, N. (2008). Interpretive biography. In J. G. Knowles & A. L. Cole (Eds.), *Handbook of the arts in qualitative research: Perspectives, methodologies, examples, and issues* (pp. 117–125). Thousand Oaks, CA: Sage.

Dlamini, B. (2006). Homosexuality in the African Context. *Agenda: Empowering Women for Gender Equity, 67*, 128–136.

Epprecht, M. (2009). Sexuality, Africa, history. *The American Historical Review, 114*(5), 1258–1272.

Florida, R. L. (2003). *The rise of the creative class: And how it's transforming work, leisure, community and everyday life*. Christchurch: Hazard Press Publishers.

Harman, S. (2016). Film as research method in African politics and international relations: Reading and writing HIV/AIDS in Tanzania. *African Affairs, 115*(461), 733–750.

Harman, S. (2018). Making the invisible visible in international relations: Film, co-produced research and transnational feminism. *European Journal of International Relations, 24*(4), 791–813.

Harman, S. (2020). The danger of stories in global health. *The Lancet, 395*(10226), 776–777.

Harnois, C. E., Bastos, J. L., Campbell, M. E., & Keith, V. M. (2019). Measuring perceived mistreatment across diverse social groups: An evaluation of the everyday discrimination scale. *Social Science and Medicine (1982), 232*, 298–306.

Jackson, A. (2015). Is 'the most homophobic place on earth' turning around? *Time Magazine (online article)*. June 1, 2015. Downloaded April 10, 2021 from: https://time.com/3900934/most-homophobic-place-on-earth-turning-around/

Johnson, C. (2019, September 24). *Trump brings up global initiative to decriminalize homosexuality at U.N. Washington Blade: Gay News, Politics, LGBT Rights*. https://www.washingtonblade.com/2019/09/24/trump-brings-up-global-initiative-to-decriminalize-homosexuality-at-u-n/

Jones, M. (2009). Phase space: Geography, relational thinking, and beyond. *Progress in Human Geography, 33*(4), 487–506.

Lewis, P. J. (2011). Storytelling as research/research as storytelling. *Qualitative Inquiry, 17*(6), 505–510.

Logie, C. H., & Gibson, M. F. (2013). A mark that is no mark? Queer women and violence in HIV discourse. *Culture, Health and Sexuality, 15*(1), 29–43.

Mavodza, C., Goldman, R., & Cooper, B. (2019). The impacts of the global gag rule on global health: A scoping review. *Global Health Research and Policy, 4*, 26.

Nhamo, M., Campbell, C., & Gregson, S. (2010). Obstacles to local-level AIDS competence in rural Zimbabwe: Putting HIV prevention in context. *AIDS Care, 22*(Suppl 2), 1662–1669.

Putnam, R. D. (2001). *Bowling alone: The collapse and revival of American community* (1. touchstone ed). New York: Simon & Schuster.

Ramon Mendos, L. (2019). *State-sponsored homophobia: Global legislation overview update.* Geneva: ILGA.

Ramsay, P. A. (2009). Claiming their own: Righting perceptions of Caribbean sexuality. *Journal of West Indian Literature, 18*(1), 86–92.

Rhodes, T. (1997). Risk theory in epidemic times: Sex, drugs and the social organisation of 'risk behaviour'. *Sociology of Health and Illness, 19*(2), 208–227.

Rhodes, T. (2002). The 'risk environment': A framework for understanding and reducing drug-related harm. *International Journal of Drug Policy, 13*(2), 85–94.

Rhodes, T. (2009). Risk environments and drug harms: A social science for harm reduction approach. *The International Journal on Drug Policy, 20*(3), 193–201.

Rutten, R. (2016). Beyond proximities: The socio-spatial dynamics of knowledge creation. *Progress in Human Geography, 41*(2), 159–177.

Semugoma, P., Nemande, S., & Baral, S. D. (2012). The irony of homophobia in Africa. *The Lancet, 380*(9839), 312–314.

Singh, J. A., & Karim, S. S. A. (2017). Trump's "global gag rule": Implications for human rights and global health. *The Lancet Global Health, 5*(4), e387–e389.

Smith, D. M. (2016). How far should we care? On the spatial scope of beneficence. *Progress in Human Geography, 22*(1), 15–38.

Solórzano, D. G., & Yosso, T. J. (2002). Critical race methodology: Counter-storytelling as an analytical framework for education research. *Qualitative Inquiry, 8*(1), 23–44.

Stewart, Z. (2017). *The legacy of British rule on LGBT rights in Jamaica and the Cayman Islands.* Master's thesis. The University of Southern Mississippi, Hattiesburg, MS. Published online by The Aquila Digital Community.

Tufford, L., Newman, P. A., Brennan, D. J., Craig, S. L., & Woodford, M. R. (2012). Conducting research with lesbian, gay, and bisexual populations: Navigating research ethics board reviews. *Journal of Gay and Lesbian Social Services, 24*(3), 221–240.

USAID. (2010). *Support to the national HIV/STI program.* USAID.gov. Washington, DC.

Weldon, S. L. (2006). Inclusion and understanding: A collective methodology for feminist international relations. In B. A. Ackerly, M. Stern, & J. True (Eds.), *Feminist methodologies for international relations* (1st ed., pp. 62–87). Cambridge: Cambridge University Press.

Chapter 3
Cultural Humility

This chapter examines the importance of cultural humility in research. It draws on experience working with Fostering Open eXpression among Youth (FOXY), an Indigenous and Northern youth sexual health program in the Northwest Territories, Canada. It begins with a reflection on research with FOXY that identified the salience of cultural humility in research. There follows a reflective conversation with Candice Lys, the co-founder and Executive Director of the organisation. Next, there is discussion of the larger value of cultural humility in offering a lens for work with Indigenous Canadian and Northern communities, and for researchers more generally working in communities they do not belong to and which have experienced histories of colonization and marginalization. The chapter concludes by looking at Indigenous approaches to knowledge and wellbeing more generally. In so doing, it invites researchers to consider the benefits of approaching research from the stance of cultural humility. Using this approach, researchers can explore both the convergence and divergence of their own approaches to knowledge with Indigenous knowledge practices, thereby identifying areas for learning and growth.

3.1 Learning Moments Working in Northern and Indigenous Communities

An acquaintance from the LGBTQ scene in Toronto reached out to me on Facebook Messenger. She told me she had moved to Yellowknife, a small city in the Northwest Territories (NWT), Canada and had begun co-organizing a local LGBTQ pride group and pride celebrations. Seeing that I was queer and working with LGBTQ people in other places in Canada and globally, she suggested that perhaps I could do some research with the NWT pride group. I hesitated as I wanted to make sure any work I did was connected to local communities and aligned to their priorities—particularly as had never been to the NWT. I had though spent a summer in Canada's

C. Logie, *Working with Excluded Populations in HIV*, Social Aspects of HIV 8,
https://doi.org/10.1007/978-3-030-77048-8_3

North as an undergraduate student in the small former goldrush town of Dawson City in the Yukon Territory, and had memories of it being very beautiful. However, whilst there I had been busy waitressing and cleaning restaurants, and while I was able to spend time in nature as I was living outdoors in Tent City,[1] I did not have the chance to learn about Northern realities. An academic colleague who conducted research in the Arctic introduced me to a doctoral student (now graduated, Candice Lys, interviewed in this chapter) who had developed an action research project as part of her work focused on youth sexual health. Candice, from Fort Smith in the NWT, had been dissatisfied with the sex education she received while growing up and decided to do something different—this was the genesis for FOXY. FOXY provides school-based workshops for adolescents using multi-media arts formats, including drama and body-mapping, to promote sexual agency, positive constructions of sexuality, and healthy sexual communication and relationships.

After connecting, Candice and I decided to collaborate on a small planning grant to build LGBTQ collaborations in the NWT. She wanted to ensure FOXY was LGBTQ inclusive, so that is where we began our collaboration. We conducted a small qualitative research project interviewing LGBTQ youth and adults, not only in Yellowknife but also in smaller communities. We experienced difficulty recruiting Indigenous LGBTQ persons, despite Indigenous people comprising the majority of NWT's population, and harnessed FOXY's existing relationships in schools and communities. I saw Candice immediately make changes based on feedback from LGBTQ communities to reflect FOXY's openness to LGBTQ persons. Based on cultural norms and expectations, FOXY's work is sex segregated. Yet feedback generated from LGBTQ youth signalled the need for gender inclusivity moving beyond the gender binary. FOXY next opened up summer retreats traditionally designed for young women to include trans and non-binary youth. Years later Candice created a parallel program for young men, SMASH (Strengths and Masculinities for Sexual Health) that was similarly trans inclusive and young trans men and non-binary persons were also welcomed.

Following this LGBTQ work, we decided to collaborate on research to help FOXY understand the impact it was having on participants' sexual health across communities in the NWT. Over the past few years there have been several key learning moments for myself in these research projects with and for Northern and Indigenous communities. The lessons learned center on the importance of culture and tradition, and the importance of context.

Understanding Indigenous cultures requires knowing the historical and continued impact of colonization of Indigenous peoples in Canada—and across global contexts. The NWT has long been notorious for having the most residential schools per capita in Canada, where Indigenous children stolen from their families were forced to attend a Catholic education. There they were forbidden to speak Indigenous languages, practice cultural traditions, and often prevented from visiting their families, in addition to experiencing horrific sexual, physical and emotional violence

[1] https://whatsupyukon.com/Yukon-communities/Dawson-City/remembering-tent-city/.

within the institutions themselves. The last schools were closed in the 1980s, thus many young people we worked with in the NWT had a parent or grandparent who had been forced to attend residential schools. This history of violence and family separation and its intergenerational effects shapes the higher reported rates of mental health problems in the NWT. The NWT has among the highest prevalence of suicide, problematic alcohol use, and sexually transmitted infections in Canada. Strengthening connection to culture and tradition can help to counteract the effects of colonization on self-worth by strengthening community connectedness and in turn promoting healing and wellbeing.

As a non-Indigenous 'Southerner' (non-Northerner) it remained key for me to recognize that I did not have the knowledge of theories or methods that should guide sexual health interventions for young Northern and Indigenous persons in the NWT. I had to put aside my experiences from other contexts and projects to listen and learn about what works for Northern youth and what decolonization looks like in practice. FOXY's work is grounded in Indigenous ways of knowing and being. Ceremony is woven into daily activities, including smudging[2] and drum circles[3] at the beginning of workshops and staff meetings. I have one beautiful memory of working with colleagues late one evening in Yellowknife after a full-day youth retreat. We sat around a long table and I was taught how to craft tobacco prayer ties made with fabric and natural tobacco to share as gifts with participants. There are multiple other ways of traditional learning embedded in FOXY's processes, including land-based retreats where youth learn drumming, beading, and papier-mâché mask making.

I had never been part of sexual health research project where the sexual health components seem secondary and the main focus is on connecting to oneself and one another in affirming ways. And it works! Our qualitative and quantitative research findings showed that not only did this approach increase HIV knowledge, but it also raised self-efficacy around condom use. The approach—focusing on connecting the person to something bigger, whether it be art or traditional practices, and not on the health issue—was a shift for me. It pushed me to let go of the traditional way in which I did HIV research and interventions and instead to trust that my colleagues know better than myself what was needed for young Northern persons to realize sexual health. I also started to consider that perhaps sexual health should not always be the primary goal, but instead the focus should be a holistic perspective on wellbeing. Another shift was understanding the cultural value of community inclusivity. Regardless of scientific perspectives on the validity of randomized controlled trial designs, FOXY was clear that they did not want to withhold any potential benefits from young people in the NWT. As a result, we continue to stress in grant applications the importance of community inclusion as a rationale for non-controlled

[2]Smudging is a ceremonial tradition among some Indigenous cultures in North America that involves burning sacred medicines such as sweetgrass, sage and cedar. For more information: https://indigenoustourism.ca/smudging-101-with-old-hands-of-the-shoshone-first-nation/.

[3]Drum circles are a ceremonial tradition in some Indigenous cultures. For more information: http://www.northernc.on.ca/indigenous/the-drum/.

study designs. Inclusivity also meant recognizing the value and worth of persons of various ages, and in our work with adolescents this meant including Elders and youth in all steps of the programming, from development through to implementation. Learning from Elders about stories, traditions, crafts and life is central to FOXY's approach to working with youth. I had never experienced this in other contexts, as I largely witnessed segregation in programming by age and youth-only spaces.

I also learned a lot about context. The NWT has a vast land area, over one million square kilometers with low population density (0.0 persons/square kilometre). Many of the communities that FOXY works in are far from Yellowknife and require driving long distances or flying on small planes. I initially pressured the FOXY team to use tablets to conduct surveys to avoid time and errors from paper-based survey data entry. However, this did not align with the needs and realities of the team on the ground who needed to travel to remote communities on small planes, already carrying arts-based supplies. The priority lay in taking what was needed to conduct the youth workshops, and paper-based surveys weighed less compared with tablets. Other contextual factors I needed to pay attention to were literacy challenges and associated with this the time available for survey completion. Structural and social inequities such as food insecurity and mental health issues can manifest in the ways that people learn and, in their experience on the ground, FOXY noted literacy challenges. This meant reducing the length of the survey, changing survey measures, and paying attention to how to make the survey more accessible. Increasing accessibility to the findings was also key. We started making short 60 second videos of our findings so as to reach youth and other community members. Understanding these larger social determinants of health, including the high cost of food and associated food insecurity and the effects of intergenerational trauma, also made us pay close attention to the ways in which we framed research questions and analysis. Exploring social and structural factors associated with mental and sexual health challenges can avoid pathologizing the youth and families in the NWT as they point to the need for systemic changes. Paying attention to context and how people navigate geography and structural barriers to education helped me to understand the need to listen and adapt to meet the needs of the place and team.

Reflecting back on events, participation in this research helped me to question my own sense of what research looks like, what rigour and strong design mean when planning a study, and what inclusivity looks like when working with communities that non-Northerners and non-Indigenous people might classify as hard to reach. It helped me to consider what decolonizing my approach to research needed to involve: centering Indigenous knowledge, culture, and values; honouring land-based approaches; and focusing on identifying social and structural inequities that are the root cause of health disparities with Northern and Indigenous youth.

3.2 In Conversation—Candice Lys

Carmen: *I am thinking about the work that FOXY and SMASH is doing in the Northwest Territories and I am wondering if you could talk a bit about what guided you into developing FOXY and SMASH. What was the inspiration?*

Candice: *I don't know that I knew what to do to create FOXY and SMASH. Coming out of my Master's degree I was just starting to get involved in research, and when I started my PhD, I really wanted to do something that had a greater impact on the North than a dissertation that was going to sit on a shelf.*

Building off what I learned in my Master's degree, I talked with young women all over the North about what they wanted to see in sex education. When I started my PhD I was initially part of a project in Greenland that I had just committed to. I went there, I met the research team and the community. I then jumped on a plane back to Canada, landed in Denmark and opened my phone. And there was a notification that my organization was receiving money from the Public Health Agency of Canada to do an intervention. I thought I better switch gears because it makes more sense for me to be home in Northern Canada. I think it is really important for folks from the North, and small and remote locations, to go back home again and work on building their own communities. So for me, it just made sense to go back home. I needed to do something that was independent, hands on, and quickly evolving, to have greater impact. Working with youth—they are fun. There is a lot that we can learn from them. As well, I had it in my mind that I struggled with a lot of things as a teenager and I wanted to do something to be who I needed when I was younger. So that is where the early, early days of FOXY came from, talking with FOXY Co-Founder Nancy. We thought, what are we going to do? Let's try something with the arts. We started working with youth and it was really fun. We kept doing it.

Carmen: *There are many things that I have noticed that are different than other research projects that I have been involved in. And one of them is that you always involve Elders. And I noticed that it has been a very central and very powerful part of FOXY, and different than other research that I have seen with youth, to bring in this wisdom of the elders. How did you decide to do that? What do you think that brings?*

Candice: *As an Indigenous person, for us it is just a no brainer that we have Elders involved in the work that we do. These are our spaces when we get together: there are young folks and adults. Of course, there are Elders. It is more surprising to me that other youth programming does not always involve Elders. And one of the things that has actually been kind of extra special, is that we have also started involving children as well. That is really important, as it is all of the quadrants of the medicine wheel. It is our youth and our elders, across from each other in the medicine wheel, as well as our adults and our babies. It is really important that we have the Elders there and we have the babies there, because it is recognizing all of these different generations and the good things that they bring to everything that we do and the lessons that we can learn from them.*

Carmen: *Another thing that stood out for me working with you has been integration of the arts in many ways, for instance with body mapping, beading. How did that come up?*

Candice: *I do not see myself as an artist and I never did. Which I think also speaks to how the arts work. The idea that I do not identify as an artist, but I still see the benefits of the arts and how they can have an impact and can be a vehicle for everything that we are doing. I think, if anything, that makes the case stronger for the arts. It is more about process than about products. It is about engaging with the arts, using more than your words to explore things, to think about things—and sometimes to not think about things—and to just be in your body. It is a way of learning that is so versatile and in a lot of ways really efficient. It is more efficient than sitting. It is more efficient to be sitting there doing something with your body and your hands than to be sitting there in front of a screen or whiteboard at a school. I think that was part of the appeal for me.*

Carmen: *I was working with African and Caribbean transgender women in Toronto. And we had this art intervention, with hearts and mirrors. And Yasmeen, who was leading this with me, said the conversations would never have happened if you just sat people in a circle and asked them to talk. The art gave them the ability to connect with themselves, sitting on their own, but together. That makes me think of the time you invited me to a national Indigenous youth meeting in a huge room with FOXY and SMASH and you were guiding everyone to do body mapping. And you asked me to make a body map as well, and it was really powerful for me to also take part. I shared that experience of what it is like to do your body map in a room with a lot of other persons working on their own together. It was an interesting feeling.*

Candice: *Yes, we try to get all of our facilitators to do body maps. Even our Elders have done their own.*

Carmen: *What is behind you wanting us to do it, too?*

Candice: *I think it is important to experience body mapping, to know how it feels in your body, to know the different things that you think about. The real purpose of body mapping is to look at internal and external resources and strengths. I think it is really helpful for everybody to take some time and to live within your body and to just focus on yourself and to focus on who you are—and the great things about yourself. Even the challenges that you struggle with. One of the unintended consequences of the COVID-19 pandemic is the idea that we have more time. Most of us at least have more time to hang out and do these things that we never have time to do. A lot more people are engaging with arts. They are doing their knitting and their cross-stitching and their painting and baking. Baking can be art. Why not? The arts can be so, so versatile. But it is doing something—it is processing emotions. The reason so many people are making bread right now is because it is helping them to process this collective trauma that we are going through.*

Carmen: *That is so interesting, particularly regarding the idea that we can be connected without necessarily having to talk to one another. With the body mapping, we are all connected and sharing an experience, but it doesn't have to look like we are just sitting and looking at each other's faces.*

Candice: *We all have unique strengths and differences in our past and present. But we are all in this room together with these bodies and these experiences and memories and strengths. There is a lot of power in that. We co-create while individually learning.*

Carmen: *There are two other things that stand out for me in my research with you. One of them is the importance of music, because I have not experienced music to be so central or so important in research before. For instance, drumming has such a large role and you create songs with youth. How do you think music is helpful in your work with youth?*

Candice: *Of all the arts, music is universal among youth—the number one art that they connect with. There are so many different kinds of music. They by no means all like the same song, although there are definite themes and songs that are hits. But music is a universal experience for young folks. The power of drum circles is that you do not have to know how to play an instrument to show up and be part of a drum circle. You can participate in a drum circle without ever touching a drum. If you are comfortable, you can pick up a drum and you can just start drumming. And even the smallest kids can drum like Luca (my son), he runs around with a little drum beating on it. He is fifteen months old and he runs around beating anything he can, pots and pans.*

Drumming is important for us for a lot of reasons. For one, traditionally in many cultures, drumming is something that's only done by men. But in FOXY, women can drum in a space because it is all women. It's a safe space for them to be able to drum together and to experience the drum. Whereas in other places, they might never have that opportunity.

Drumming—there is the beat of the drum. Every culture in the world has a drum of some kind. It is a heartbeat of communities. If you take a baby to a drum dance, almost all of the babies are asleep because it is that common heartbeat. Drumming uses bilateral stimulation in the brain. It is a way to process trauma, because you are using both sides of your brain in active drumming. Drumming can be connected to ceremony and to really important conversations.

I do not know if I have talked about how drum songs come about. But in the teachings that I have received, drum songs are not written. They are caught. We believe that all of the songs are actually out there in the universe. And when you do a ceremony to catch a drum song, if you are lucky enough to do that, that is you catching one that's already out there. Being given the ability and the permission to share that song with others is amazing. Catching a drum song is a really powerful experience.

Carmen: *What I have learned a lot from you also is the importance of making the time for tradition, including smudging, and that also reflects how you weave in connecting with the land in the Peer Leader Retreats. You integrate not just humans, but also non-human elements of the world, like animals, trees, nature. How do you think that helps you connect with youth?*

Candice: *There is something about being out on the land. It is just good for the soul, it is good for you taking young folks out on the land. That is what we try to do every opportunity we can. We try to get them out of Yellowknife, out of the city,* *because the whole perspective of everything shifts as soon as you are out on the land. There feels like there is more time. There is more opportunity to connect with yourself and with others and to slow down and to focus on these really important things. Somehow taking youth out on the land opens up this way of communicating with youth that just is not possible when we are in the big city. It shifts perspectives and it shifts priorities, and it makes you feel more connected to yourself and to others. There is a lot of humility that comes with being out on the land. You need to be humble, you might feel like you are king of the castle in the city, but when you are out on the land you need to know what you are doing to be safe. You need to realize that the elements and other animals and everything that is out there is so much bigger than just you.*

Carmen: *How do you draw those connections between taking youth out to the land and sexual health? Because you are successful at addressing multiple dimensions of health with young people, including improved confidence and sexual health. You are able to use these different elements of nature, tradition and music. All of these different things we have been talking about. What you do is different than most approaches that are not working with Indigenous communities in the North. You have this unique lens that may also be beneficial to other people and other places.*

Candice: *I think the strength of being out in the land is that you are better connected to yourself and better connected to others. The land helps you to reflect on relationships because you are in a relationship with the land. It helps you to reflect on all kinds of relationships, including your relationship with yourself, relationship with partners, with family, and within your community. Being on the land is a catalyst for reflection.*

Carmen: *Why do you think that young people love FOXY and SMASH so much? Why are you so successful at reaching young people from many communities and engaging them?*

Candice: *Well, one of the reasons is that we involve youth in everything that we do every day. We work with youth to develop things, implement them, and everything we do is peer led. It is co-led with the younger folks on our team as well as the adults on the team. We have three or four times as many youth on staff as we do have adults. And it is really important to have youth to co-develop leadership and to be the connectors with the young folks, because I am in my thirties—I am a mom. When I started FOXY, I was younger. I was twenty-eight, but I was still a long way away from thirteen or fourteen.*

It is really important to have those younger folks who can be the role models, the mentors, and understand that they make mistakes, too. That is part of mentorship, to be able to make a mistake and move on. I think that is really important that our young folks model for us.

Carmen: *And what does mentorship look like in in FOXY and SMASH?*

Candice: *In every opportunity they are doing something to help out the younger folks. Sometimes that means leading a workshop. Sometimes that means sitting one-on-one with somebody who might be struggling and just wants to have a chat. They are up there teaching sex ed and they are sitting with youth and meeting with them. Every opportunity that they have—young folks are always watching. It is not helpful* *to create a rule, for instance, you are on the clock from 3:00 p.m. to 5:00 p.m. Because you are always being watched and observed and they are always learning. It is the littlest thing, it is conversations that they have one-on-one. It is bringing our Elder tea, asking her if she needs anything and bringing it to her. I love the young folks who work for us. They are all awesome. And I learn so much from them.*

Carmen: *I notice that you give the opportunity for youth to move up in order to become more involved in FOXY. For instance, some of the people who were participants are now peer leaders and you have long term engagement. You also are very clear on your values. For instance, when putting in a grant, now I have stopped asking you, but at first I suggested that we offer FOXY to some communities and then not to others in order have a control group. You felt very clearly that we value giving everybody FOXY that we possibly can, and you want to share this opportunity as wide as possible. I have noticed that this feels intentional.*

Candice: *It is definitely intentional for us. It is about trying to include everyone and to create a space where everyone is welcome. We are not perfect at it, but we try.*

Carmen: *I really love that. Going back to your discussion of mentorship, what I have noticed is that you and all of the peer leaders are role models to the wider community everywhere you go, even when you are not on the clock. For instance, I know that with your FOXY sweatshirts, you ask people to avoid drinking alcohol when you are wearing this because you are a symbol in the community. I think that is really powerful that people can walk around knowing that if they are wearing this sweatshirt, that they reflect these larger values.*

Candice: *Yes, they are ambassadors for our programming. They are one piece of a huge movement. For us it is important that if you are wearing our FOXY or SMASH t-shirts or hoodies that you are not using alcohol or other drugs or smoking while our logo is present. It also speaks to our value that regardless of who you are, we still love you and we still want you to be part of us. It is not us saying, "no, no, no, you can't drink. You cannot smoke pot". It is us recognizing that we still love them and still want them to be part of us. But turn your hoodie (sweatshirt) inside out. Still keep FOXY and SMASH close to your heart, but recognize that other people are always watching. We are trying to create a movement here, and it is important to try to recognize and respect that.*

Carmen: *I have a question pertaining to the theme of this book. What do you think when people say that adolescents are hard to reach?*

Candice: *Never before in all of our history has a group of people, adolescents, been so connected. And in some ways easier to reach, as they have grown up with cell phones in their hands. When somebody says that young folks are hard to reach, I think often perhaps people are not going about it the right way. Young people don't have time for bullshit and if they are not into something, either they will tell you or they will shut you out because it is just not their priority. If you are not able to reach them, sometimes it might be genuine connectivity issues like in the North it can be really hard to have Internet. It is not that I do not want to communicate with you, it is that this system is not allowing me to. But that might mean that you are not able to reach them once or twice, here or there. More often, it can be that they have no* *interest in connecting with you. Perhaps you need to go back to the drawing board and figure out what is not working.*

Carmen: *This leads to my next question: what would you like to say to the next researcher who wants to work in the North or a Northern community with youth, maybe with Indigenous youth? What is your advice?*

Candice: *Is it a researcher from the community or not?*

Carmen: *Let's give two examples. One, they are from the community. One, they are not. First, let's say they are from the community.*

Candice: *If you are from the community, speak with community members, figure out what they want, what they need. That is always important. Recognize that when you are coming from your community, you are the experts of your community, regardless of whether or not academia granted you a degree. For researchers who are coming from outside of the community, I think the most important thing is recognizing humility, recognizing that you are not the experts in the community. That everything that you do should reflect the needs and the wants of community members rather than trying to impose any kind of research questions or methods or to check that box on grants. It is about building genuine relationships with communities and being ready to support communities in whatever way that they want, including to not engage with you.*

Carmen: *That is amazing. When you say humility, what does that look like?*

Candice: *From a research perspective, humility includes recognizing that you might know a lot about some things, you might have a lot of experiences, but that does not mean you are the expert in anything. You are the expert in nothing. Even if you have a PhD, like I do in public health, I am still learning every day. I am still being humble. Being humbled is to take your lessons as they come, to learn from Elders, to recognize that there is so much we can learn from babies. To recognize also the limits of academia. That we are always learning and we are always being humbled, because sometimes we are wrong and we need to own our mistakes. We need to allow ourselves that space to be uncomfortable. It is not easy sometimes, especially as an academic, to be uncomfortable and to feel like you do not know stuff. But I think that is really important as a researcher.*

Carmen: *I am so grateful that you took the time to share all of this. I am glad you brought up the notion of cultural humility.*

Candice: *Sometimes it is called cultural safety. I like the notion of humility, though. I prefer it because it is about recognizing where you fit within structures. I do not think this is reflected in other terms, I hate the term cultural safety.*

Carmen: *I actually feel as if the term cultural safety is referring to something different. It makes it seem as if I need to be safe, as if I need to put on a seatbelt. It is not asking you to consider your position as not being the centre. It is making you the protector, whereas actually I can be the harm if I do not watch myself.*

Candice: *Humility implies self-reflection, whereas cultural safety and cultural competency do not. How can we be culturally competent in anybody else's culture? It also overlooks the diversity within cultures.*

Carmen: *I agree, I think humility is more about asking questions of yourself and self-reflecting. Humility also implies that not everybody has to tell you the answers.*

You cannot just walk into wherever and have folks tell you the answers because you want them.

Candice: *Exactly. Especially, a lot of Indigenous cultures and a lot of our teachings are these lessons that you have to figure out for yourself and that you do not just automatically get the answer to. You need to figure it out.*

Carmen: *I love that: as researchers we need to take the time and thought to figure things out. Something that I was so impressed with and wanted to reflect on was widening your circle. When we first started working together, a lot of what we were working on was around how to be more inclusive of LGBTQ people. And you really did a lot of work on that. And then it became thinking of how to widen the circle to include boys and men and, other trans folks. I wanted to mention that I think that is such a huge gift that you have given to communities in this thoughtful expansion. Is there anything you wanted to share about how you made those decisions?*

Candice: *With FOXY, we were started by two cisgender women. Because we started with what we knew and with our own experiences. I think it was important to recognize that what we knew was conditional. Like for myself, I am cisgender, I am heterosexual, and I am also not a dude. I think it is really important to find ways to be more inclusive. Yet also recognizing that I do not have those answers about how to be more inclusive of LGBTQ folks, because I am not part of that community. I could not just find those answers myself because I did not know what the answers were. I also do not think it would be right for me to universally make decisions about what the needs are for young men or for LGBTQ folks or any anyone else. None of us have these universal experiences to be able to speak for everyone. It was really important to be able to do that research and to talk with folks about what they needed and what they wanted to see, rather than just imposing stuff and hoping for the best, which goes back to the cultural humility piece as well.*

3.3 Applying a Cultural Humility Approach and Learning from Indigenous Approaches

> Cultural humility is a lifelong process of self-reflection and self-critique whereby the individual not only learns about another's culture, but one starts with an examination of her/his own beliefs and cultural identities (Yeager & Bauer-Wu, 2013, p. 2).

Cultural humility, a key concept that emerged in the reflective conversation with Candice, refers to the ongoing practices of self-reflection and learning that are central to engaging in genuine and respectful relationships, including conducting research with persons who may have different lived experiences based on wide range of factors, including race and ethnicity, gender, sexual orientation, geography, ability and socio-economic status (Tervalon & Murray-García, 1998; Yeager & Bauer-Wu, 2013). As discussed in the above quotation, it requires a continuing examination of the assumptions, biases and values developed in one's social world and through lived experiences. The concept of cultural humility has its recent origins in medical training the USA. It implies a commitment across the life course, a process of active engagement, and a relational practice with oneself, communities, service users, research participants, and colleagues (Tervalon & Murray-García, 1998).

Central to cultural humility is the dynamic, heterogenous, and multi-dimensional nature of the cultures that exist across place, including home, family, work, and spiritual centres. A core element of cultural humility is that a person should focus on themself and their own environment, personal values, beliefs and culture(s) before trying to understand someone else's life, culture or worldview (Yeager & Bauer-Wu, 2013). Cultural humility includes taking action to transform power imbalances in relationships between oneself and others, including between the researcher and study participant. Such actions may include developing partnerships that are mutually beneficial and advocate for community social justice goals. Here, I want to examine the role of cultural humility in preparing researchers to work respectfully with communities, and then focus on Indigenous approaches to knowledge and wellbeing. Applying these frameworks together can inform respectful and social-justice oriented research.

3.4 Conceptualizing Cultural Humility

Researchers' lack of knowledge and understanding of the lived experiences of communities they are working with can contribute to practices that reproduce racism, LGBTQ stigma, sexism, among other forms of stigma and discrimination. The concept of cultural competence was initially developed to tackle these knowledge gaps (Tervalon & Murray-García, 1998). Yet the premise underlying the term *competence*, as defined by the Merriam-Webster dictionary, includes "the quality or state of having sufficient knowledge, judgment, skill, or strength". This implies that one can reach a point at which enough knowledge and skills are acquired regarding culture. It also assumes culture is static and cultural knowledge is finite (Tervalon & Murray-García, 1998). The gaze of cultural competence is usually outwards with a focus on learning about the 'other'. This outward gaze overshadows the need for inward reflection to acquire self-knowledge (Tervalon & Murray-García, 1998; Yeager & Bauer-Wu, 2013). In addition, the framing of culture as static may result in stereotyping, overlooking cues that provide insight into nuanced lived realities. Another limitation of a cultural competence framing is its tendency to conflate culture with ethnicity and race, thereby missing diversity within cultures as well as the intersection with other factors including gender, sexual orientation, socio-economic status and geographies. This reflects Candice's observation about the need for self-reflection in a cultural humility approach that may not always be found in cultural competence framings. A competence framing also focuses on the researcher's education and needs in order to be confident and equipped in order to help; this reinforces hierarchies over who holds knowledge and who needs to be assisted.

In contrast to cultural competence, cultural humility views culture as dynamic. Rather than focusing on confidence and competence, cultural humility can provide the researcher with information on how to respect and understand culture in ways that improve the experiences of marginalized communities in and beyond research (Yeager & Bauer-Wu, 2013). This focus on humility suggests that as we undertake lifelong learning about cultures other than our own, we recognize what we do not know. Such a perspective maps onto Candice's discussion above about the need for humility: "humility includes recognizing that you might know a lot about some things, you might have a lot of experiences, but that does not mean you are the expert in anything. You are the expert in nothing." This recognition demands that researchers embrace courage and flexibility as they undertake self-critique and self-reflection, and approach practice and research as learners rather than experts (Tervalon & Murray-García, 1998; Yeager & Bauer-Wu, 2013).

Learning from a stance of cultural humility extends beyond knowledge acquisition to self-awareness and attitudinal change. As researchers we should explore our personal, professional, and research values that underpin our life and our research first, before engaging in research (Tervalon & Murray-García, 1998; Yeager & Bauer-Wu, 2013). Viewing the ways in which our own cultural identities are multi-dimensional and evolving over time can help us expect the same for other cultures. Reflecting on our profession requires considering how our identities and worldviews are shaped by professional codes of conduct—that themselves are embedded in institutional cultures with biases and blind spots (Yeager & Bauer-Wu, 2013). Social work, for example, has an ongoing history of aiding the colonization and destruction of Indigenous families, historically through support for residential schools and schooling, and currently through child welfare systems that disproportionately separate Indigenous families in Canada (Blackstock, 2007). Western conceptualizations of health and healing dominate health professions and suppress other ways of knowing and being, including approaches that incorporate land, spirit, and traditional knowledges as central to wellbeing.

Examining values around research, knowledge, and ethics can shape the ways researchers conceptualize questions and proposals, and how data is analyzed, interpreted, and shared. Scientific values, such as the 'gold standard' of randomized controlled trials that I discussed with Candice earlier in this chapter, may conflict with community values of inclusion and access to research benefits. The questions that are asked, if not inclusive of cultural strengths and values, can perpetuate cultural stereotypes (Yeager & Bauer-Wu, 2013). Changing institutional norms about research can also mean changing who is considered a researcher and who is a participant. Researchers can examine whether the research team—including decision makers—reflects members of the community the research is in service to.

3.5 Developing Cultural Humility

Cultural humility requires mindfulness, relationship building, and understanding history. Mindfulness encourages noticing, and self-knowledge about bodily cues, thoughts, emotions and awareness of context and other dimensions of the environment (Yeager & Bauer-Wu, 2013). The core of mindfulness lies in recognizing when thoughts and emotions arise, and it is through this space that one can become aware of biases and judgment. Candice mentioned that one of the aims of the arts-based body-mapping method is to provide space for reflecting on who you are, including your struggles and strengths. Humility requires flexibility, humbleness, and identifying and deconstructing stereotypes and biases. It also involves actively working to reduce power imbalances between researchers and participants, including when identifying priorities, methods, and knowledge sharing. Seen from this perspective, the researcher no longer needs to be the expert, as it is their role to listen and learn from participants (Tervalon & Murray-García, 1998).

An understanding of history, and specifically histories of colonization, slavery, and medical mistreatment, is key for researchers who want to practice cultural humility. For instance, learning about the history of family separation and residential schools, and the current mistreatment of Indigenous children and families in child welfare systems, is needed to contextualize people's lives and understand that mistrust of researchers and persons in positions of authority is rational and warranted. The historical and recent forced sterilization of Indigenous women in Canada (IJRC, n.d.) and other global contexts, and overrepresentation of Indigenous peoples in Canadian prisons (Government of Canada, 2016), are other valid reasons why Indigenous peoples mistrust non-Indigenous researchers and systems. These historic and current inequities create valid reasons for mistrust and for choosing to disengage from research, whereby people may intentionally become hard to reach to avoid processes and systems that perpetuate harm.

Applying community-based research approaches can also help with learning and practising cultural humility. These involve working closely with communities to understand the contextual factors that shape health and wellbeing, addressing community-identified priorities, building on community resources and adaptive strengths, and partnering with local community groups and agencies (Tervalon & Murray-García, 1998). Research can also prioritize building lasting relationships with, and creating positive impacts for, participating communities, including applying principles from action research to advance social justice goals (Datta, 2018). This action focus reflects Candice's inspiration for becoming a researcher: "I really wanted to do something that had a greater impact on the North than a dissertation that was going to sit on a shelf." Researchers can support how knowledge is translated to benefit communities, including in ways that can be understood by non-scientists such as videos, infographics, and policy briefs (Ford et al., 2016).

The practice of cultural humility can help researchers to understand their own knowledge gaps regarding Indigenous epistemologies, and to recognize diversity within and between cultures. Cultural humility can be a first step to starting a research journey, including building trusting relationships. Research with Indigenous communities can involve researchers locating themselves: who they are, where they are from, and why they are doing this research (Lavallée, 2009; Loppie, 2007). Cultural humility and its implications for conducting research can encompass such issues as community protocols, collective data ownership, relationship building, approaching communities with a focus on strengths, and collective knowledge gathering and sharing (Datta, 2018). It also reflects the need for flexibility and continued reflection on the research process and alignment with community priorities (Ford et al., 2016).

3.6 Centering Indigenous Knowledge

Five elements of Indigenous knowledge, frameworks, and epistemology may be helpful for researchers engaging in ongoing self-reflection as part of the practice of cultural humility. These elements, also discussed by Candice, are applicable across the research process and include: decolonization and the use of Indigenous research protocols; respect for Indigenous approaches to knowledge and theory; recognition of the importance of medicine wheel teachings; the value of land-based knowledge; and concern for love and reciprocity.

3.6.1 Decolonization and Indigenous Research Protocols

Decolonization aims to center Indigenous land, people, sovereignty, and ways of being and knowing the world (Denzin, Lincoln, & Smith, 2008). Applying this approach to research can be transformative for both the researcher and participant in alignment with social justice goals (Datta, 2018). Understanding Indigenous research methods can facilitate research processes that are appropriate, caring, and respectful. Researchers may have different responsibilities when working with Indigenous communities (Datta, 2018), such as respect for cultural (not only research) protocols, for instance regarding the giving and receiving gifts, data ownership, sharing meals, and leaving a positive impact on the community. There are no pan-Indigenous approaches to knowledge paradigms and protocols, (Lavallée, 2009; Loppie, 2007) so the examples that are provided here come from Indigenous researchers largely based in Canada with the caveat there is diversity and nuance and specificities within and between Indigenous cultures. The research example in this chapter with FOXY also involves young people living in Northern Canada of diverse Indigenous cultural backgrounds, including First Nations, Métis and Inuit. The goal of examining decolonization and Indigenous knowledge frameworks is to consider how this knowledge can help researchers examine their research approach, inspire self-reflection, and identify gaps in knowledge that need to be addressed.

3.6.2 Storytelling, Theory, and Sources of Knowledge

How knowledge, values and theory are approached and understood may differ between Indigenous and Western, Euro-American and Euro-Canadian perspectives (Loppie, 2007; Simpson, 2014). Across diverse global contexts, Indigenous peoples have shared intergenerational cultural and historical knowledge conveyed using oral traditions such as storytelling (Loppie, 2007). Knowledge, philosophies, and socially congruent practices and behaviours are shared by Elders using stories, myths, and legends. Stories can be used to share theories across generations, from babies and children who may focus on understanding the literal meaning, to youth and adults who understand more metaphorical meanings and seek to apply the principles to their life (Simpson, 2014). Elders teach in ways that show how the meaning of stories changes across the life course, while still positioning themselves as learners. Stories may make reference to traditional codes of ethics, with their own epistemology, pedagogy and metaphors (Simpson, 2014). As Candice put it, in "a lot of Indigenous cultures and a lot of our teachings are these lessons that you have to figure out for yourself and that you do not just automatically get the answer to." Storytelling is one such approach; stories are adapted to the context and life situation to help persons engage in problem solving and decision making. Storytelling is dynamic and can shift over time to reflect changes in society (Loppie, 2007).

Other Indigenous principles relevant to research include recognition of the existence of multiple sources of knowledge. Expanding beyond only cognitive approaches to understanding, Indigenous research methods include a focus on dreams, intuition, memories and implicit learning (Loppie, 2007). These sources have been described as the intertwined elements of empirical observation, traditional teachings, and revelation (Lavallée, 2009). Empirical observation includes multiple perspectives across contexts, for instance when learning about plants' medicinal properties (Lavallée, 2009). Traditional teaching includes sharing knowledge across generations. Understanding Elders as knowledge holders (Datta, 2018; Lavallée, 2009), as discussed by Candice, reinforces the importance of researchers engaging with Elders for guidance when working with Indigenous communities—irrespective of the age of study participants. Researchers should treat Elders as valuable sources of knowledge, ceremonies, knowledge, stories, and cultural practices. Revelation, or spirit, as a source of knowledge includes learning from dreams, visions and intuition. This includes *blood memory*, or the process whereby persons learn from ancestors through blood lineages. This spiritual element of knowledge is not measurable or observable. Western research training promotes the idea that researchers 'discover' knowledge, create concepts and ideas, and should try to observe or measure phenomena to understand them –such training strongly conflicts with perspectives that knowledge is passed down through ancestors, blood, spirit and dreams (Datta, 2018). Candice provided the example of working with youth in drum circles to catch a song, as all songs already exist in the universe. These three sources of knowledge (observation, teaching, spiritual) are interconnected and equally important in

Indigenous knowledge systems. Researchers should consider how their research might explore these multiple sources of knowledge.

3.6.3 Harmony, Balance, and Medicine Wheel Teachings

Relationality and the connections between people, nature, and land, and the physical-mental-emotional-spiritual dimensions of people, comprise elements of Indigenous epistemology (Lavallée, 2009). Loppie (2007) described how this value of holism elicits an understanding of a person and all elements of their life: *individuality*, including agency and freedom; *relationality*, comprising commitments to oneself, one's community, the environment and cosmos; and *harmony and balance*, including respect for the sacredness in life, humans, and non-humans. From this perspective, research cannot be objective due to the interconnectedness of people—including the researcher and participant—as well as the connectedness between emotional and mental processes that are used in the process of conducting research.

The medicine wheel, as described by Candice in our reflective conversation, is used as part of Indigenous teachings to reflect these principles of harmony and balance (Lavallée, 2009). The medicine wheel is a circle that reflects the infinity of life with four quadrants that are separated and interconnected, and with colours that may differ by Nation (Lavallée, 2009). The four quadrants reflect wholeness and balancing, including: physical, mental, emotional, and spiritual domains of wellbeing; family, community, environment and earth; directions (North, West, South, East); and/or can reflect four races (African, Asian, Indigenous, and white) (Dapice, 2006; Lavallée, 2009). Working with the medicine wheel can provide a holistic approach to wellbeing and health that considers cyclical knowledge, such as seasons, rather than only linear understanding (Walker, 2001). Indigenous pedagogical approaches also seek to integrate medicine wheel dimensions: see it (physical), know it (mental), feel it (emotional), and do it (spiritual) (Wallace & Ambridge, 2012). Indigenous researchers have also applied the medicine wheel to research practices. For instance, the East (spiritual) dimension could involve researchers considering the ways that they are connected to research participants and communities. The South (emotional) dimension could remind researchers to work from a place of authenticity and from the heart. The West (physical) includes the embodiment of knowledge, and in this dimension researchers can examine their personal relationship to nature, self, others and traditional cultural teachings. Finally, the North (mental) dimension of the medicine wheel can foster research that balances intellectual pursuits with wisdom and research to produce harmony and balance in participating communities (Walker, 2001).

3.6.4 Land-Based Knowledge

Indigenous values and knowledges also center land-based knowledge and learning. Integrating knowledge of and connection to land, history, animals, and plants can produce research experiences that align with community priorities. Practices such as hunting reflect historical and current knowledge of climate and land: "to 'go hunting' requires the collaborative knowledge of generations who have signalled where moose and other animals like to be in specific times of year, how they move, and how they are impacted by snow or water conditions and temperature" (Ballantyne, 2014). In a related vein, Wildcat and colleagues describe how:

> Spiritual healing and grounding is an important benefit that comes with cultivating a strong relationship to land. This is more than a fortunate by-product of engaging in land-based practices. Teachings and practices based in spiritual values are critical components of learning and teaching on the land. Protocols that demonstrate respect and reciprocity, such as putting down tobacco, making offerings, ceremonies, or particular ways of harvesting or treating unused animal parts, are a part of Indigenous land-based education (Wildcat, McDonald, Irlbacher-Fox, & Coulthard, 2014, p. 10).

These protocols also include the burning of sacred plants such as sage or sweetgrass before an event or ceremony referred to as smudging (Lavallée, 2009), which is practiced by FOXY during team meetings, training events, and peer retreats. The smoke shared in smudging practices is used to cleanse a space, objects, and people (Lavallée, 2009). In Canada's North, climate changes have deeply impacted communities, including by changing permafrost thaw patterns which in turn change the ability to travel across the land safely, alter the diversity of wildlife and plans, and transform the quality of water and food. These changes particularly impact individuals, households and communities in the NWT that engage in subsistence-based hunting and land use (Ford et al., 2016). Such changes have resulted in rapid adaptation, signaling the importance of Northern Indigenous communities' knowledge of how to protect land and resources through community networks and resilience (Ford et al., 2016; Ratelle & Paquette, 2019). Sustainable and contextually relevant adaptations to climate change center traditional knowledge, local customs, cultural norms and values, community ownership and decision making (Ford et al., 2016)—while also acknowledging the structural determinants of adaptation, including poverty. Researchers should recognize and value the adaptation skills and protective factors persons employ to adjust to climate change, as well as larger structural constraints—including colonization and inequities—and the ways these factors converge to shape health and wellbeing. While the land provides opportunities for reflection it is also a teacher regarding how to safely manage the natural elements to survive. In this way, and as Candice described, there is "humility that comes with being out on the land" that can spark reflection on relationships with the land, self and others.

3.6.5 Love and Reciprocity

Approaching research with Indigenous communities, among other communities, involves a process of building empathic, compassionate relationships of care. Candice described how this caring inspired her to start FOXY: "I wanted to do something to be who I needed when I was younger." The concepts of care and reciprocity are important components of Indigenous epistemologies. Elsewhere Simpson has described how:

> In addition to the land (including the spiritual world), the context for Nishnaabewin is profoundly intimate ... Gaa-izhizhaawendaagoziyaang requires love, the word zhaawen, a part of the word Gaa-izhizhaawendaagoziyaang, means to have complete "compassion for another in one's thoughts and mind. It has a connotation of bestowing kindness, mercy, and aid. It includes ideas of pity, empathy and deep unconditional love" (CBC, 2014; Simpson, 2014, p. 10).

Research that does not recognize and respect these values can produce harm, and researchers may find it challenging to engage people, and could possibly consider those persons hard to reach. Knowledge and meaning from Indigenous worldviews are produced in the interdependent relationships between people, nature and animals (Simpson, 2014). Relationships can also reflect processes of reciprocity (Ford et al., 2016). Loppie (2007) has described how group discussions with Indigenous women provided the chance for story sharing and reciprocal learning. Young people offering mentorship to other youth and serving their Elders is another example of the reciprocity that is central to FOXY's work. As Candice described it: "in every opportunity they are doing something to help out the younger folks ... It is the littlest thing, it is conversations that they have one-on-one. It is bringing our Elder tea, asking her if she needs anything and bringing it to her." This example also reflects multi-generational reciprocity.

Reciprocity also includes making offerings to the land before taking a harvest, to animals after hunting, and to Elders (Simpson, 2014). Offerings of tobacco or other gifts demonstrate respectful caring and mutuality. The crafting of tobacco ties I discussed earlier in this chapter reflected these concepts, whereby we created offerings to show gratitude. In this process of creating these offerings we also strengthened relationships and shared traditional teachings of creating tobacco ties for ceremony. Lavallée (2009) discusses reciprocity as central to research aligned with Indigenous frameworks. This reciprocity can be multi-level: participants' knowledge is a gift to researchers, while the opportunity to share perspectives and have voices heard in the research process can be a gift to participants, and the honoraria and/or offerings provided to participants are also symbols of respect and gratitude.

3.7 Rethinking 'Hard to Reach' Through the Lens of Cultural Humility

In sum, as researchers we can position ourselves as lifelong learners, while also taking the initiative to learn as much as we can about the legacies of colonization and the structural and socio-environmental factors that perpetuate social and health disparities. Cultural humility can be a guiding framework so researchers can look inward to identify their own cultural values and traditions first, and then learn about the dynamic, diverse and adapting cultures of the communities we want to engage with. Relationship building can be central to this practice, as communities will identify priorities for research and what role (if any) they want you as a researcher to play. The importance of connecting with communities was a salient recommendation by Candice for researchers, when she said: "everything that you do should reflect the needs and the wants of community members rather than trying to impose any kind of research questions or methods".

Researchers working with Indigenous communities and in contexts they do not belong to should adapt and plan for potential challenges to practice cultural humility and learn from Indigenous approaches. This may cause tension with academic expectations and structural constraints. For instance, time and skills are needed for collaborative and community-based research, and the researcher cannot rush the process. Long term funding is required to sustain and grow relationships and acquire the resources needed to effect change, and obtaining these resources will require creativity, commitment and patience.

Moving forward, as researchers grounded in practices of cultural humility we should remain flexible and open to change research directions as needed, and accept our own failures in the research process when we do not get it right—even question the concept of right (Loppie, 2007). As Candice described in our conversation earlier in this chapter, researchers need "to recognize also the limits of academia. That we are always learning and we are always being humbled, because sometimes we are wrong and we need to own our mistakes. We need to allow ourselves that space to be uncomfortable." These challenges also signal how researchers need to be able to accept 'no' if communities decide not to participate in research. Research may not always be beneficial or wanted, even if the researcher practices cultural humility and employs a community-based research approach.

For research to contribute to Indigenous goals of self-determination and social justice goals more generally, researchers should build skills and capacity to ensure that the research products themselves are useful and relevant for communities. There is a chasm between the creativity embedded in Indigenous knowledge and Western approaches to science disciplines (Loppie, 2007). Producing research that is uplifting, and honouring the strengths, adaptability and wisdom of communities—rather than solely focusing on health challenges—can help to dismantle the stigma and negative stereotyping directed towards Indigenous communities. In turn, strengths-based research can contribute to processes of empowerment. Being available, self-reflective, and vulnerable in the research process can result in the researcher paying attention to what is most important and valuable to Indigenous and other communities. As Candice explained: "Young people do not have time for bullshit and if they are not into something, either they will tell you or they will shut you out because it is just not their priority." When researchers are authentic and self-knowledgeable and the research is germane to communities, they will be far less likely to struggle to reach persons.

References

Ballantyne, E. F. (2014). Dechinta Bush University: Mobilizing a knowledge economy of reciprocity, resurgence and decolonization. *Decolonization: Indigeneity, Education and Society, 3* (3), Article 3.

Blackstock, C. (2007). Residential schools: Did they really close or just morph into child welfare. *Indigenous Law Journal, 6*(1), 71–78.

CBC. (2014). *Fragile freedoms: Indigenous love, law and land in Canada's Constitution*. Canadian Broadcasting Corporation. http://www.cbc.ca/player/Radio/Ideas/ID/2440345608/.

Dapice, A. N. (2006). The medicine wheel. *Journal of Transcultural Nursing, 17*(3), 251–260.

Datta, R. (2018). Decolonizing both researcher and research and its effectiveness in Indigenous research. *Research Ethics, 14*(2), 1–24.

Denzin, N. K., Lincoln, Y. S., & Smith, L. T. (Eds.). (2008). *Handbook of critical and indigenous methodologies*. Thousand Oaks, CA: Sage.

Ford, J. D., Stephenson, E., Willox, A. C., Edge, V., Farahbakhsh, K., Furgal, C., Harper, S., Chatwood, S., Mauro, I., Pearce, T., Austin, S., Bunce, A., Bussalleu, A., Diaz, J., Finner, K., Gordon, A., Huet, C., Kitching, K., Lardeau, M.-P., . . . Sherman, M. (2016). Community-based adaptation research in the Canadian Arctic. *WIREs Climate Change, 7*(2), 175–191.

Government of Canada. (2016, August 5). *Statistical overview on the overrepresentation of indigenous persons in the Canadian correctional system and legislative reforms to address the problem—spotlight on Gladue: Challenges, experiences, and possibilities in Canada's Criminal Justice System*. Government of Canada Department of Justice. Ottawa.

IJRC. (n.d.). *Forced sterilization of indigenous women in Canada*. International Justice Resource Center. Retrieved June 10, 2020, from https://ijrcenter.org/forced-sterilization-of-indigenous-women-in-canada/

Lavallée, L. F. (2009). Practical application of an indigenous research framework and two qualitative indigenous research methods: Sharing circles and Anishnaabe symbol-based reflection. *International Journal of Qualitative Methods, 8*(1), 21–40.

Loppie, C. (2007). Learning from the grandmothers: Incorporating indigenous principles into qualitative research. *Qualitative Health Research, 17*(2), 276–284.

Ratelle, M., & Paquette, F. (2019, December 2). Climate policy should reflect the resilience of northern Indigenous communities. The Narwhal, Victoria.

Simpson, L. B. (2014). Land as pedagogy: Nishnaabeg intelligence and rebellious transformation. *Decolonization: Indigeneity, Education and Society, 3*(3), Article 3.

Tervalon, M., & Murray-García, J. (1998). Cultural humility versus cultural competence: A critical distinction in defining physician training outcomes in multicultural education. *Journal of Health Care for the Poor and Underserved, 9*(2), 117–125.

Walker, P. (2001). Journeys around the medicine wheel: A story of indigenous research in a Western University. *The Australian Journal of Indigenous Education, 29*(2), 18–21.
Wallace, A., & Ambridge, S. (2012). *Full circle: First Nations, Métis, Inuit ways of knowing: a Common threads resource*. Toronto: Ontario Secondary School Teachers' Federation.
Wildcat, M., McDonald, M., Irlbacher-Fox, S., & Coulthard, G. (2014). Learning from the land: Indigenous land based pedagogy and decolonization. *Decolonization: Indigeneity, Education and Society, 3*(3), Article 3.
Yeager, K. A., & Bauer-Wu, S. (2013). Cultural humility: Essential foundation for clinical researchers. *Applied Nursing Research, 26*(4), 251–256.

Chapter 4
Critical Hope

This chapter reflects on the process of developing a research project entitled *TRANScending Love*, with African, Caribbean and Black transgender women in Toronto, Canada. It begins by describing the process of developing the project, and the way that listening to community priorities resulted in a redirection of research purpose and methods. This is followed by a reflective conversation with Yasmeen Persad, the co-principal investigator and community leader. Subsequently, I examine the literature on critical hope and self-compassion to understand the importance of these concepts in research focused on people such as African, Caribbean and Black transgender (trans) women who experience social exclusion and are often labelled hard to reach.

4.1 Learning from Work with Transgender Women of Colour in Toronto, Canada

I had been working with an African, Caribbean and Black AIDS service organization in Toronto for a decade, and we had recently completed a successful HIV prevention program with African, Caribbean and Black (henceforth referred to as Black) young cisgender women. I came across an intervention for African American cisgender women that was classified as evidence-based on the US Centers for Disease Control (CDC) website, and it had included the training manual and protocol. We held a focus group with young Black cisgender women in Toronto, and they shared with us their feedback and ideas to tailor the content for their context. There was enthusiasm in the room, and participants called for us to make the intervention open to sexually diverse women, to bring in Canadian specific HIV statistics, and to include information about African and Caribbean HIV epidemics alongside HIV in Canada more generally. We left inspired and made these adaptations to the training manual. The intervention, called *Healthy Love*, was implemented in a range of community-based

C. Logie, *Working with Excluded Populations in HIV*, Social Aspects of HIV 8,
https://doi.org/10.1007/978-3-030-77048-8_4

agencies across Toronto. It was so well received that the collaborating African, Caribbean and Black AIDS service organization decided to integrate it into their HIV prevention program. They applied for and received funding from the City of Toronto to mainstream *Healthy Love* into their regular programming for young Black women.

Healthy Love, however, was focused on the lived realities of cisgender Black women. While we could tailor it to include sexually diverse women, after talking with AIDS service organization staff we knew we needed a different approach for Black trans women. Not only might Black trans women have increased HIV knowledge in comparison with cisgender women, but they also experience social exclusion rooted in transphobia that presents unique barriers to HIV prevention (and healthcare more generally). Finding the *Healthy Love* program on the CDC website had been so helpful, I later searched for other trans specific interventions. I next encountered *T-SISTA* (Trans Sisters Informing Sisters on Topics of AIDS), an HIV prevention program for trans women of colour. We thought this seemed like a good program to adapt for Black trans women in Toronto. It was strengths-based and included poems by, and interviews with, trans women of colour in the USA. We hired a trans community leader in Toronto as the research coordinator with decades of activism and service provision experience with trans women of colour.

The first step we took, as we had done with *Healthy Love*, was to elicit feedback regarding *T-SISTA* from Black trans women. To do this, we held a focus group at a community agency serving sex workers. When we started talking, focus group participants made it clear they were not interested in hearing or talking about HIV prevention. They explained they were fed up with hearing about HIV, and knew about it already. They told us we also needed to shift the focus away from trans women's bodies to the larger context of their lives. One woman asked us: "how can we love ourselves in a world that hates us and wants to kill us?" Another described how researchers needed to focus on self-love, as self-love was key to people feeling worthy of engaging in HIV preventive practices. Participants were tired of the dominant focus on trans women's sexual practices, and wanted research that focused on their hopes, dreams and whole lives. I felt worried about what to do next, as my plan for adapting the *T-SISTA* intervention for the local Toronto context had been rejected. I needed to switch gears to focus on self-love—something I had never considered in the research context.

Working closely with a team from the African, Caribbean and Black AIDS service organization and two trans women community leaders in Toronto, including Yasmeen Persad interviewed in this chapter, we created a new plan. I started Googling 'self-love' activities, entered the world of Pinterest, and presented a few options in consultations with the team. Body mapping, an activity I had included in research with women living with HIV and with Indigenous youth in Northern Canada, was vetoed as it focused too much on the body. Trans women were tired of having the research gaze focusing on their anatomy. Sexual objectification of trans women's bodies is pervasive. We decided on three arts-based activities to form the workshop that community leaders named *TRANScending Love*. The first took the form of an anatomical image of a heart. Participants were encouraged to write inside of the heart the names of the emotions that blocked the arteries. In the ventricles coming out of the heart, they were asked to draw and write down coping strategies. The second activity involved a hand-held mirror on which to write messages of self-love using glass markers. Finally, we shared blank affirmation cards printed with the words 'you are loved' and on which participants could write affirming messages to one another, and to other trans women.

We held three *TRANScending Love* workshops, each in a different location, to reach diverse trans women of colour. The first meeting was held in a LGBTQ community centre, the second in a Black AIDS service organization, and the third in a sex worker drop-in centre. We were surprised at how well the activities were received. Initially we expected to give people the option to take part in one of the three activities, providing craft supplies for each activity on separate tables. Yet participants across workshops wanted to do each activity, moving from table to table. At the end of the workshop, we invited members to share with the larger group their anatomical heart, mirror messages, and affirmation cards. This became a deeply emotional process. Participants' discussion of the mirrors, in particular, included stories of navigating pathways from loneliness and loss of friends and family following their gender transition, to a new sense of hope through connecting with other trans women. In story after story, we heard similar trajectories from loneliness to finding community. When sharing their anatomical hearts, participants identified a range of coping strategies for navigating difficult emotions—including sex, art, cooking, music, friendships, and reading. Each participant finished their turn sharing by reading from their affirmation cards and then placing them in a large jar. The affirmations were overwhelmingly about strength and overcoming current challenges; some declared that trans women are beautiful and that things will get better. In one message that stood out for me, a participant had written and then crossed out the word 'beautiful' in the phrase 'you are beautiful' to read 'you are strong'.

After the workshops we held a community event to invite some participants to be part of a panel presentation. We enlarged the images of the anatomical hearts and affirmation cards to display around the room, and printed decks of *TRANScending Love* cards. Nearly a hundred people came, and we were surprised by how much these messages of love, coping and self-acceptance resonated with them. Following this, we presented the cards and the process at various World AIDS Day events, HIV conferences and forums, and eventually to AIDS service organizations and health centres. My involvement with our team in *TRANScending Love* presentations ended following the shift from sharing research findings to informing service provision. I recommended that agencies hire and support trans community leaders from our study to share *TRANScending Love* findings. After finishing *TRANScending Love* and publishing a paper detailing the research process (Logie et al., 2019), I was unsure what to do next. How innovative and important would funders consider a self-love and self-acceptance intervention in HIV research? The plastic mirrors and arts-based materials were not environmentally friendly. Working with small groups of women had been successful, but how could we scale this up across various contexts? At the same time that I was unsure about moving forward, I also realized how important this focus on self-love, acceptance and sharing affirmations had been not only for participants but also for myself as a researcher. Until then the narrative underpinning much of my work has centered HIV and explored barriers and facilitators to engaging in HIV prevention and care cascades. Moving HIV to the side to focus on journeys to self-love felt new to me, but also necessary if we listen to trans women about what most matters, and their decision making regarding engaging in health promoting practices.

Reflecting on lessons learned from *TRANScending Love*, many moments stand out. The first of these was awareness of my feelings of disappointment when what I thought was a great idea was not what focus group participants were interested in. In fact, participants were not interested in the entire focus of the grant—HIV. This reminded me how essential community engagement is, and how researchers need to remain flexible and creative. A second learning moment occurred in the same focus group when participants asked for researchers in general—and me in particular—to consider and address how trans women can love themselves in larger contexts of social and structural exclusion. As an HIV researcher I needed to grapple with participants' call for the focus to shift away from trans women's sexual practices, sexual risks, and bodies. It might be expected that I would be better equipped as a social worker to explore self-love than colleagues trained in biomedical or clinical practice. But I was at a loss and needed to start from the ground up. Body-mapping, an arts-based method I had experience with, was also not well suited to working with trans women. As a result, I was challenged to find new research frameworks and theories. At the end of each focus group we asked participants about their experiences with the workshop process. Participants described the arts-based activities helped them to document their journeys toward self-acceptance and strategies for navigating daily survival. Individual experiences reflected a collective narrative. In this way the workshops provided a forum for trans women of colour to build connections and solidarity, in turn fostering hope. As one participant shared: "It is breathtaking to know that you can find trans women who would before knowing anything else about you, be open to share their stories, and be open to give you support" (Logie et al., 2019, p. 41). In the end, narratives from *TRANScending Love* participants signalled the importance of HIV researchers focusing on the interconnections between the intrapersonal processes of hope and self-acceptance, and relational processes of connection with trans community, that provide a foundation for navigating contexts of social exclusion and health-related decision making.

4.2 In Conversation—Yasmeen Persad

Carmen: *In HIV research, whole groups of people are called hard to reach. The theme of this chapter is on the importance of critical hopefulness, which is hopefulness in contexts of social injustice. I wanted to talk to you because I thought that TRANScending Love (T-Love) was for me, the most powerful research I have ever* *done about the need for hopefulness. I want to start off by asking you how you feel when people call trans communities hard to reach?*

Yasmeen: *I am tired with the language of 'hard to reach'. It is the way that service providers and the researchers and the people who want to work with trans persons always seem to have probably not the right objective. You are not using the right approach to try to reach trans people. And I think it goes back a lot to trust if you are not, like I am, connected to trans women. It is just something for work. Ask yourself, 'what are my own personal biases?' Researchers and service providers and folks who want to do focus groups and all of these interactions with trans people tend to forget that for so many years I have seen experiences of trans people's exploitation. They are not providing a very welcoming environment and people can feel very misunderstood. A lot of people feel really vulnerable in research, so then they step back.*

Carmen: *What do you think are some of the approaches that do not work?*

Yasmeen: *In general, people come out of the blue and say "hey, I want to work with trans people on ..." Really? We do not know this person from nowhere. And most of the time the research team has no trans persons. I know where trans women are located, where we are. They have never accessed or been part of the community like I was, even as an ally or anything to that effect. And then out of the blue, for example, they would send me an email or mail me a package of stuff saying "hey, could you distribute this to trans people?" Literally, this approach is so wrong. I may have met you once, but that does not give you the opportunity to say, "hey, do this." They have to build a relationship. There has to be some relationship building before we can start to get involved or invite folks and say, "OK, we are ready to do this research."*

Carmen: *Working with you, we were doing the focus group for TRANScending Love and I thought we were simply going to adapt this HIV intervention T-SISTA and it was going to be great. And then we got a lot of pushback because people said, "You need to focus on self love. You need to focus on how people can love themselves in this world that is so tough". It really struck me because I had never heard anybody say that to me before—focus on self love. It actually started me thinking so much more about love and hope in research.*

Yasmeen: *Researchers and people coming in think they know what we need to know. They underestimate the knowledge that trans people have about themselves and their access to services in the community. And a lot of that ties in with the stigma around trans people and marginalization. People may be thinking "Oh, my, these poor trans people did not get care. They do not access HIV care, STIs, all these different things." And then as you probably know from that conversation, we know about HIV, we are tired of hearing about STIs. We want to talk about ourselves. We want to talk about our experiences of being newcomers or refugees, of being an immigrant, living in poverty, stuff that people do not tend to think of that is much more important to us than medical care.*

Carmen: *For me, I personally felt so moved when we did the Transcending Love workshops. I felt a lot of hope, watching people connect to themselves in a different way that was really loving and also with one another. I felt there was a lot of* *connections and kindness and hope, and that change is possible and we can be part of that change.*

Yasmeen: *I am learning that in using an arts-based approach it can bring out something in people that would not have come out in a focus group, for example, if we sat around and had pizza and asked persons to talk about self-love. But giving people something visually to work with, something that was really simple, it was so deep for a lot of people. The mirrors and the heart maps, people felt really connected. The participants still think about that and talk about it. You could have something like that every three months. People would really come to it because it is strengths-based, it is not disease focused. It takes away from that stigma. There are so many negative statistics out there, figures of how much trans women of colour are more likely to be affected by HIV. Some stuff is real. But sometimes it feels a bit too superficial. We are not only HIV or we are not only sad people, but we have a life that is not bad!*

Carmen: *One thing I noticed that I would love to get your thoughts on is that people shared their journeys to accepting themselves. And I felt like every single workshop we heard the same kind of trajectory, from one of pain and loneliness with rejection to one of self-acceptance and how that happened through community. I felt as if there are all these hopeful journeys from pain to not saying it is perfect, but to a place that was better.*

Yasmeen: *I think part of it, though, was so powerful because this particular population that we worked with (transgender women of colour) often do not get that space to talk about self-love and to talk about acceptance of who they are. There is no space like that. Just to be in that space, with African, Caribbean and Black trans women is to feel that there are more people like me. They are just not around as much in the community. There are a lot of trans women of colour that do not ever come out to events. You realize that there was a need.*

Carmen: *Another thing I was really moved by were the affirmation messages that people wrote to each other, the messages of love.*

Yasmeen: *Yes, the way the system is set up it pushes us against each other sometimes. The way they all came together and wrote those really affirming messages, people understood. I think afterwards that population specifically really connected with each other on a different level that they would not necessarily have.*

Carmen: *I feel so grateful that I was part of that. What do you think about hope? I have been thinking about how important it is for researchers to truly believe that things can get better and that people can make their lives better and each other's lives better.*

Yasmeen: *The hope is often there, but researchers' language that they use might not reflect an approach of hope. It does not come across as though you are asking people about hope or what is hopeful for them. It could feel like it is an evaluation of a group of trans people, not that we want to talk about hope or what is helpful for you. I understand how these words do not have a lot of strength versus if we say, "oh, let's do our research project and measure this." Researchers, service providers, everybody who seems to want to do the work with trans people have to* *engage in that hopeful language, in those kind of conversations in order to reach people in ways that say, okay, now you are speaking to us and not about us.*

***Carmen:** Through this journey you have been sharing TRANScending Love all over Canada. What was that experience like for you?*

***Yasmeen:** It was amazing. It is always amazing to just share it and talk about it. People were really, really open to adapting it across different spaces. You know, we shifted out of the box to something like this that is quite simple but moving and could really change people's lives in a very special way. It also changed me after being in that group, because I have not been in such a space with so many trans women of colour in a long, long time. Some groups may include one or two trans women of colour. But I have never been in a group of twenty-five. I think that has made people trust me more and feel connected to me more. I still connect with a lot of them that I had met for the first time in the workshops.*

***Carmen:** How much of this experience do you think is because of the content being about self-love and hope? Do you think the connection that you felt with people would be the same if it was just about HIV?*

***Yasmeen:** It was the topic. Because I have done other HIV and sexual health focus groups, and this was different. I do not think the connection was made as deep as this.*

***Carmen:** This workshop also made me also think about myself. It is not just that these research participants need self-love, I also need self-love. There is this human need to be connected to yourself and others. After TRANScending Love you and I made a video series*[1] *together that you envisioned focusing on the lives of newcomer (immigrant) trans women of colour. What are your hopes for that?*

***Yasmeen:** It just happened to be that this awesome group of people came together. When we started to film and reflect on the topics and what we really wanted to cover, we could really be ourselves and we did not have to be fake or talk with an accent. It was really organic and natural. I hope with what we are trying to say, people get it, and it comes across as a teaching and learning tool for a lot of people. We also have a TPOC (trans person of colour) cookbook that is almost finished. We thought it would be awesome to launch the cookbook and videos together. It is not going to be a little launch. It is going to be a red carpet in a ballroom. Both the videos and cookbooks are celebrating trans persons of colour. We want to make it a celebration, because it is just too much sadness and depressing stories on a day-to-day basis. We want to celebrate that evening and say, look, we did some great, amazing work for this population.*

***Carmen:** I want to know the role you think celebration plays in helping us in the struggle for social justice. Why do we need to celebrate?*

***Yasmeen:** Well, we need to celebrate for many reasons. We need to celebrate because the people we work with give us that motivation to go to work and to work*

---

[1]The video series hosted by Yasmeen Persad on health needs and priorities of trans women of colour can be found on YouTube (https://www.youtube.com/channel/UCH7_yna3dHYGCkLgJCBAKGw/videos) as well as the SSHINE Lab website: https://sshinelab.com.

even harder. We know if we celebrate people's lives we can show them that it is not only about hardship. You are going through this rough thing, but there are parts of you and things that you are doing that are amazing. We are also celebrating the representation we want you to see. We want you to see yourself and reflect and celebrate. I think that is one of the approaches that really could work.

Carmen: *If we do not have hope when we are fighting for equality, we are going to run out of fuel.*

Yasmeen: *We need to take a moment to celebrate so we do not burn out too. You cannot keep going, going, going on until burnout. No. We get a moment to celebrate when you feel like you cannot keep going, and then you can start again. There is some force that keeps us going. We need to get the work done, because people need the support.*

Carmen: *When I present on TRANScending Love I talk about the idea of hope to researchers. People are kind of surprised, but they are open and I think they like that message.*

Yasmeen: *Absolutely. I do a lot more presentations now and I can tell people there is hope, despite what I have just told you about challenges facing trans people whereby everything seems so dark and dreary with so many barriers. There is hope, there is love and resilience. Sometimes I notice they also seem shocked. I think we can really get caught up in the academia part of it and forget the human side of it—at the end of the day these are human beings. We are talking about real people with real feelings and real hopes, real goals—everything that we have, dreams. And we have to bring it back to that. Not just numbers and stats and figures.*

Carmen: *When I went to your TPOC cooking group, it was so joyful.*

Yasmeen: *You should see what it has grown into. It is twelve to sixteen people on a weekly basis. All are trans women of colour. I did not know what to expect. Oh my! They come back, they volunteer and make friends. It has just been amazing.*

Carmen: *Why do you think this TPOC cooking group is such a success?*

Yasmeen: *Because there was a huge gap. There was nothing like it. This is no way to live where African and Caribbean trans women and other trans women of colour have nowhere to go where we feel that we belong. I hate to say it, but that is the reality of it. When you see people like yourself, where you are reflected, then you feel that this is a space where I belong. It started off as a way to talk about sexual health. And now you should see the kind of things we are doing and talking about. People come up and celebrate their birthdays. We support them with housing and clothing, support around violence. It has morphed into an unbelievable experience. We teach people new recipes and give them food that they can take home to cook. It has just really been something. With the word-of-mouth people just keep coming and coming.*

Carmen: *I hear so much happiness in your voice.*

Yasmeen: *A couple of weeks ago, one of the participants, because of her living situation, cannot live fully as a trans woman. So we celebrated her birthday. One of the peers did her makeup, we pitched in and supported her with getting on her wig and a dress. And it was such a cheerful moment to see her. She could be in a space where she could really be herself. The peers really helped her and showed her how* *to do her makeup. We got a cake. And this is why I do the work I do. It was one of those moments where you really create joy and community.*

Carmen: *This is my last question. This book is for researchers. What do you want to tell them?*

Yasmeen: *I think, of course, they mean well. When we do this research and we start thinking about how we are going to apply for a grant for this particular research question and this particular population, they do mean well. I think where some of the challenges come in, is that they do not necessarily connect a lot with the population. They might always have the sort of 'research hat' on, or the 'academia hat', where they think, "oh, this particular population needs this kind of research." They are going to do this research just because they know the topic, but deep down they are not doing it from their soul. Perhaps they should say "Okay, let me step back and think about my role in this. What exactly am I as a researcher? What type of approach will I be using in how the research is done? And when the research is finished, how will this impact this particular population?" And again, researchers need to think about the human aspect of it, these are people we are going to be researching and these are people's life stories. We are going to go deep down and we may trigger all kinds of stuff. Are we really ready for that? How are we going to make the changes needed together with the population? Then the research can be so powerful.*

Carmen: *I appreciate what you said about the need for researchers to look in their soul, not just in their minds.*

Yasmeen: *That is why our research has been successful, because we have tried to keep the people still involved in many ways. We will come around and ask, what are we doing that works? What are we not doing? And they see spinoffs of various research projects. Like TRANScending Love was a spin-off into TPOC cooking in a way, and that was a spin off into the video series on trans women of colour. When they see the videos they know, again we are here, and we are going to make change in a different way.*

Carmen: *The stories of hopefulness are really shifting the perspective away from illness.*

Yasmeen: *I think so. You have had so many years of experience with research. I think the way you are going to put this book together, hopefully new researchers and people who have already been in research will get a wake-up call. They can really think about this hopeful approach they need to do this work with. We need more lenses. We talk about intersectionality and we need to look at this from a new lens, perhaps the intersectionality of feelings and emotions. People can be pushed to the sides of society, but you have to be hopeful or else it would be easy to give up.*

4.3 Applying Critical Hopefulness and Self-Compassion to Advancing Research with Socially Excluded People

> Hopelessness paralyzes us, immobilizes us. We succumb to fatalism, and then it becomes impossible to muster the strength we absolutely need for a fierce struggle that will re-create the world. I am hopeful, not out of mere stubbornness, but out of an existential, concrete imperative. I do not mean that, because I am hopeful, I attribute to this hope of mine the power to transform reality all by itself, so that I set out for the fray without taking account of concrete, material data, declaring, "my hope is enough!" No, my hope is necessary, but it is not enough. Alone, it does not win. But, without it, my struggle will be weak and wobbly. We need critical hope the way a fish needs unpolluted water (Paulo Freire, 2014, p. 2).

The above quotation by Paulo Freire encapsulates the elements of hopefulness that reflect the lessons learned in the preceding reflection and dialogue about research with trans women of colour. By building connections with the communities they wish to work with, and applying hopeful, strengths-focused, and creative approaches, researchers may find that socially excluded persons may not be so hard to reach after all. Critical hopefulness refers to the need for hope in the struggle for social justice and equality. It involves developing critical awareness of social justice issues in tandem with creating constructive resolutions. Critical hope is a necessary ingredient in being able to transform reality—but it is not enough on its own. Also required is self-compassion which orients the researcher toward recognizing suffering and pain as a shared human experience. Engaging people with acceptance, kindness, and patience when undergoing challenges encourages awareness of our common humanity as people who share the experience of pain and make mistakes. It also provides opportunities for marginalized communities, and for marginalized communities and academics, to work together in solidarity to advance social justice.

Historically hope has shaped affected communities' responses to HIV. Herbert de Souza's "The Cure of AIDS" poem poignantly describes the hope that he dreamed would come with a cure to HIV: "suddenly, I realized that all had changed because there was a cure. That the idea of inevitable death paralyses. That the idea of life mobilizes … even if death is inevitable, as we all know. To wake up knowing that you are going to live makes everything in life meaningful" (de Souza & Parker, 1994, p. 48). Simon Watney (2000), in his book "Imagine Hope: AIDS and Gay Identity", describes how among people living with HIV, hope was an essential component of healing. Yet at the same time hope is precarious. Watney (2000) describes something of the challenges of hope before the advent of highly active antiretroviral therapy: "Hope? Hope for what? Of course you hoped, but it was very dangerous. If you hoped for too much you were bound to be disappointed. If you expected very little, you might even possibly be admirably surprised" (p. 263). In a different vein, Barnett, Seeley, Levin, and Katongle (2015) approach hope as a factor central to the response to HIV in Uganda. Their study found that hope was associated with (a) structural factors, such as owning a home and land; (b) agency generated from having supportive family and friends; and (c) having an optimistic attitude toward life. These different examples signal how over a fairly long period of time, across cultural contexts and among diverse communities and populations, hope has helped people to think about how to respond to HIV and AIDS.

Against this background, this chapter will explore the concepts of critical hope and self-compassion to understand how these approaches can enrich our research and provide insight into the TRANScending Love case study presented earlier.

4.4 Hope and Critical Hopefulness

4.4.1 Understanding Hope

Hope has been shown to be associated with improved wellbeing, psychosocial and physical health (Snyder, Lopez, & Pedrotti, 2015), including in longitudinal studies (Ciarrochi, Parker, Kashdan, Heaven, & Barkus, 2015). Defined in many ways, hope has been described as a cognitive process that can help persons reach their goals (Snyder, 2000). Cognitions central to hope include agentic thinking, whereby persons believe they can do something, and pathway thinking, through which people develop action plans to reach their goals (Weis & Speridakos, 2011).

Herth's (2000, 2001) multidimensional approach to hope examines the ways in which people strive for future goals while managing health issues and other stressors. It includes several different dimensions: cognitive-temporal, such as the belief that one can achieve a goal; affective-behavioural, having confidence in an action plan to reach a goal; and affiliative-contextual, comprising social, spiritual and community support. Hope may also be understood as an emotional state that balances both confidence and uncertainty (Miller, 2007). Farran, Herth, and Popovich (1995) likewise conceptualize hope as multidimensional, comprising the experience of human life as challenging, a spiritual component rooted in faith, thought processes that consider goals in the context of available resources, and relational processes whereby hope is influenced through interaction with others (Farran et al., 1995). Relational dimensions of hope include sharing, feelings of care, and belonging (Miller, 2007). Feeling accepted and understood by another person can inspire hope. Conversely, inequitable power relationships with healthcare providers, friends and family, among others, may pose a threat to realizing hope.

Hope building strategies informed by the cognitive approaches described above include community building with collective sharing of the ways in which courage and optimism are revealed in personal challenges and struggles (Herth, 2001). Yet meta-analytic findings have revealed only small effect sizes in the relationship between the hope enhancement strategies implemented in individual and group therapy and outcomes of increased hope (Weis & Speridakos, 2011). The authors suggest possible explanations. Perhaps hope is not very malleable. Or perhaps the techniques of storytelling and goal setting employed in such strategies were not effective. Other more collectivist-oriented hope inspiring strategies include a focus on: experiences, such as sharing humour, creativity, and storytelling; spirituality, encompassing meaning-making and religious practices; relationship building, including through increased social interaction and communication; and rational thought processes, for instance rethinking goals (Miller, 2007). During end-of-life care, strategies to maintain hope include recalling meaningful memories, feeling valued and accepted, generating inner peace, and providing a legacy for others.

Healthcare workers have hope that their patients' health and wellbeing will improve. They also know that hope can be healing and contribute to wellbeing. At the same time, their patients will experience hopes and fears. And healthcare providers need to be wary of instilling 'false hope' so as to not disappoint patients about their prognosis (Van Hooft, 2014). This can create a double bind. The healthcare provider can inspire hope by sharing new possibilities with the patient and addressing uncertainty (Van Hooft, 2014) regarding future hopes and fears. The HIV researcher may find themself in a similar situation of needing to consider tensions between hope and reality, yet may not have acquired experience and understanding of how to do this well.

4.4.2 Pedagogies of Critical Hope

> Without a minimum of hope, we cannot so much as start the struggle. But without the struggle, hope, as an ontological need, dissipates, loses its bearings, and turns into hopelessness (Freire, 2014).

The conceptualizations of hope described above using cognitive frameworks, healthcare provider experiences, and in (largely ineffective) hope building interventions, miss a number of key ingredients found in perspectives on *critical hope*. Freire's conceptualization of *critical hope* is rooted in an ontology of hope as necessary for political struggles for social justice. Critical hope encompasses both cognition and affect, but is a whole-body experience that includes emotions, hope, intuition, and thought (Freire, 2007; Freire & Macedo, 2003). Every person has hope—it is part of the human experience. However, instead of focusing on teaching or delivering hope to people, Freire perceived the goal of education as one of helping persons to stir hope up and extract it from within. Hope is both a social and individual phenomenon and integral to the work of an educator—and I would argue to our role as researchers. For Freire, hope is fueled by our own awareness that we are incomplete beings. Having hope signifies the search for improvement, and this in turn means we are open to learning. Despite hope being central to educational pedagogy, Freire advanced a critical perspective on hope that he distinguished from false, naïve, or simplistic hope. Freire's hope aimed to support struggles against discrimination, inhumanity, and alienation and aligned with liberation theology (Webb, 2010). While critical hope aims for humanization it is always under threat from socio-political forces creating oppression and division.

Freire saw critical hope as a radical and powerful force with the potential to change history and challenge limits, to recreate the world (Freire, 1972). Freire situates the educator's role as both patiently guiding hope toward humanization and, when needed, taking action motivated by passion and rage to challenge oppression.

This reflects his approach to critical hopefulness as one that encourages that "the impatiently patient wait" (Freire, 1972, 2007). Viewed from such a perspective, critical hope is not impatient itself but an active and thoughtful struggle for justice which at times required "just rage" and anger (Webb, 2010). Freire's conceptualization of critical hope as transformative requires both risk and aiming for an ostensibly utopian dream. Transformative hope requires personal and collective dreams of transcending the current situation to inspire action (Freire, 2007), and has inspired historic social change movements against slavery and the Vietnam war (Van Hooft, 2014).

Hope has also been conceptualized as a virtue (Van Hooft, 2014). Freire's (2016) approach to hope likened hope to love, trust, peace, humility, courage and patience. He situated hope (and pedagogy) within social and historical contexts that aimed for moral goodness to make the world more ethical and a better place (Freire, 2004). The purpose of hope, and education, is to become consciously present and aware that we are all unfinished 'works in progress'. Hope thereby "becomes a necessary component of one's existential experience, of one's radically being a presence in the world" (Freire, 2004, p. 100). Such an approach emphasizes the possibility of change, even in the most difficult of situations. As a virtue, hope can be practiced by acting courageously and generously, and such actions will guide us toward goals of happiness, connection and justice.

A cornerstone of critical hope is that it does not solely apply a critique of problematic socio-political structures, but it also offers a way forward. Webb describes how Freire's critical hopeful approach reflects "a precarious hope which moves beyond open-ended critique and emphasizes the necessity of transforming society in light of the liberating utopia" (Webb, 2010, p. 337). This type of hope can inspire new ways of practice to advance social justice and nurture approaches for persons to realize their own goals and contribute to a more just society. Freire (2004) described his utopian hope as simultaneously denouncing the current situation while announcing a better reality. In this way, the hope for justice co-occurs with critique of social inequities (Van Hooft, 2014). Christens et al. (2013, 2018) applied a multilevel empowerment analysis to better understand critical hopefulness.

Cognitive dimensions of empowerment comprise understandings of the ways in which social power operates to inform individual and collective action for social change at socio-political levels. With respect to application, Christens et al. (2013) found that only a minority of persons (7.5%) in a study of advocacy organizations in the USA were both critical *and* hopeful. In a subsequent study with secondary students in the USA, Christens, Byrd, Peterson, and Lardier (2018) reported that 15.7% were critical and somewhat hopeful while 10.8% reported being critical and exceptionally hopeful. These studies point to the need for strategies that increase awareness of social inequities while simultaneously building feelings of empowerment and socio-political agency. Such a study offers a stark reminder of how hard it is to balance both awareness of injustice and hope. Christens et al. (2013, 2018) suggest that community building, activism, organization and support can be valuable vehicles for fostering hope and action in the face of injustice.

The feminist scholar bell hooks similarly has discussed the ways in which collective efforts may spark social transformation and points to the need to share successful strategies for social change. This sharing can generate the hope needed to continue our efforts to challenge oppressive systems. hooks, like Freire, underscores the need to move beyond cynicism by developing constructive resolutions to social inequities:

> There have been many quiet moments of incredible shifts in thought and action that are radical and revolutionary. To honor and value these moments rightly we must name them even as we continue rigorous critique. Both exercises in recognition, naming the problem but also fully and deeply articulating what we do that works to address and resolve issues, are needed to generate anew and inspire a spirit of ongoing resistance. When we only name the problem, when we state complaint without a constructive focus on resolution, we take away hope. In this way critique can become merely an expression of profound cynicism, which then works to sustain dominator culture (hooks, 2003, p. xiv).

Like Freire, hooks approaches critical hope as part of radical social transformation and as central to pedagogy. Her perspective presents hope as political, with the goal of transforming consciousness and effecting change in lives (both within and outside of academia). To realize such change, hooks emphasizes the need for theory to be inclusive and accessible, rather than esoteric and academic.

Hope is empowering and can fuel educators, researchers and others working for social justice. Playing a central role in building community (hooks, 2003), hope fosters connections between educators as well as between educators and students that reflect a "liberating mutuality" (hooks, 2003, p. xv). Experiencing inequalities can produce confusion and despair. Bonds of solidarity, community, trust, and care can be forged in social justice work guided by love. Bearing witness to bonds of affinity, sharing a passion for social justice, and searching for joy can foster hope in communities of resistance. It can also help to develop individual and collective awareness of *interbeing* in community (hooks, 2003). Building such connections requires confronting and addressing our own biases, for example, toward trans women of colour. Openness to being changed can create space for hope and possibility. hooks describes the need for imagination in work to realize new visions of wellbeing, and the importance of "the space of the possible where we can work to sustain our hope and create community with justice as the core foundation" (hooks, 2003, p. xvi).

Hope can also be a verb, linked closely to a particular event or episode, and hopefulness can be framed as a personality characteristic or a quality of experience (Van Hooft, 2014). hooks discusses the way in which teaching from a pedagogy of hope can be joyful, as can be working in communities of resistance grounded in hope. Others extend this linkage between hopefulness and joy to larger ways of experiencing the world: "Hopefulness is an essential ingredient in joyfulness. To live life with joy is to be able to project the promise of a hopeful future for oneself and for others" (Van Hooft, 2014, p. 52). From this perspective, hopefulness is a pathway to individual and collective happiness.

Participants' narratives in our research with trans women of colour reflect these notions of critical hope, in which pain, inequity and marginalization were discussed alongside the belief that things can improve. A *TRANScending Love* participant's description of her mirror reflected this hope and her wish to share this hope with others: "My mirror is just 'love' and 'it'll be better'. I feel like a lot of people start off very rocky and it's good to remind you that things get better. So, that's my message to my younger self and also to any other person who wants motivation." Another participant's description of her anatomical heart reflected the way in which pain and suffering can contribute to growth and a better future:

> The leaf [drawing] represents growth. There were a few things in my past that, at the time they felt very, very hard on me, and I wondered why they were happening. But when I sit back and look at those things, if those things didn't happen, I wouldn't be here today, and I wouldn't be who I am. So, every time I encounter a struggle now, I don't see it as something bad, because I just look forward to what this struggle is going to bring in the future.

A critical hopeful perspective approaches pain and struggle resulting from marginalization, such as the racism and transphobia experienced by trans women of colour, as challenges that can be confronted and contribute to future growth. *TRANScending Love* participants, particularly in their affirmation cards written for other trans women, reinforced the messages that things will improve. In this way personal and collective goals for living authentic, joyful and connected lives as trans women were supported by a perspective that balanced awareness of stigma, injustice and suffering with the belief in a better future.

4.5 Self-Compassion

In her book "Teaching community: A pedagogy of hope", hooks (2003) describes how: "we are connected in our suffering. That connection is part of our understanding of compassion: that it is expansive, that it moves in a continuum" (p. 159). This perspective aligns with the central tenets of self-compassion theory. Here, compassion refers to the ability to be open to hearing about, and being moved by, the pain and suffering experienced by someone else and, in turn, experiencing emotions of kindness and a willingness to help to reduce pain (Neff, 2003).

Compassion also implies approaching other's failures and mistakes with non-judgment and an understanding that mistakes are part of the human condition. When expanded to include oneself, self-compassion applies the same acceptance and non-judgment to oneself and one's own pain, mistakes, and failures, and situates these experiences within the context of the larger human condition. Applied by Neff (2003) to understand psychological wellbeing as an alternative to self-esteem, self-compassion has roots in Eastern philosophical thought, particularly Buddhism. Self-esteem is an individualistic construct focused on comparing oneself to others and to normative socio-cultural expectations. Self-compassion, on the other hand, refers to treating oneself with kindness, care and support.

There are three central components to self-compassion: "self-kindness vs. self-judgment, common humanity versus isolation, and mindfulness versus over-identification" (Neff & Knox, 2017, p. 1). Self-compassion theory is unique in psychology as it moves beyond ideas that people are self-centred to instead consider that persons are often the most unforgiving and hostile toward themselves. Focusing on oneself as being worthy of compassion can have a ripple effect whereby this compassion and concern is extended toward others. Self-compassion can nurture feelings of interconnectedness with others and, in turn, this interconnectedness can promote feelings of equality, dignity, and respect toward others.

While concerns have been expressed that too much of a focus on self-compassion may lead to inaction, it may in fact motivate actions for change that are guided by patience, kindness and gentleness. A lack of compassion for oneself may inspire inaction and reduced self-awareness. Neff (2003), for example, has argued that "the care intrinsic to compassion should provide a powerful motivation force for growth and change" (p. 87). Self-compassion can inspire actions to improve wellbeing for both oneself and for others.

There is an important distinction between self-compassion and self-pity. Pity is an emotion that implies disconnect from others and a distinction between issues that are one's own and those of others. Pity is predicated on separateness rather than feelings of interconnectedness. Perhaps this is why in our reflective conversation Yasmeen laughed when she said "things are not so bad" for trans women, as researchers may presume with their singular focus on the problems they face. Instead, Yasmeen recommended cisgender researchers start to view trans persons as humans—with the same shared challenges, hopes, dreams, and goals as researchers themselves. Developing self-compassion provides the opportunity for researchers to understand the interconnectedness between themselves and persons labelled hard to reach as people who share the same hopes, suffering, and dreams.

Mindfulness is an approach to self-compassion which encourages the person to sit with and observe pain without overidentifying with it. An expansive, flexible, and nonjudgmental perspective on pain can generate richer insight into challenges. The opposite of mindfulness and self-compassion is resistance to pain, which in turn may lead to further suffering and loneliness. Mindfulness, self-kindness, and feelings of interconnectedness interact. Mindfulness can facilitate self-kindness by reducing attachment and identification with one's suffering, and may nurture feelings of interconnectedness by helping contextualize suffering as part of a shared human experience (Neff, 2003). Self-kindness and feeling connected with others can help to provide perspective on life challenges, in turn enhancing mindfulness. Feeling connection with others and being aware of the shared nature of pain and struggles, can help to engender self-kindness and self-forgiveness. hooks (1989) describes how experiences of suffering from oppressive contexts can produce hopelessness and despair, yet sharing these struggles can also produce possibilities for solidarity and resistance. She describes how a space of marginality is:

> much more than a site of deprivation, that it is also the site of radical possibility, a space of resistance. It was this marginality that I was naming as a central location for the production of a counter hegemonic discourse that is not just found in words but in habits of being and the way one lives. As such I was not speaking of a marginality one wishes to lose-to give up or surrender as part of moving into the centre-but rather as a site one stays in, clings to even

> because it nourishes one's capacity to resist. It offers to one the possibility of radical perspective from which to see and create, to imagine alternatives, new worlds. This is not a mythic notion of marginality. It comes from lived experience (hooks, 1989, p. 20).

From this perspective hooks views the pain of marginalization as a place of opportunity to connect with larger efforts towards resistance. Importantly, such a perspective shifts the focus away from giving up a marginalized identity to seeing it as a space for change and possibility.

Significant health benefits derive from self-compassion. In two meta-analyses, self-compassion has been shown to be strongly associated with psychological and subjective wellbeing and emotional resilience: lower stress, anxiety, negative affect and depression, and increased happiness, positive affect and life satisfaction (MacBeth & Gumley, 2012; Zessin, Dickhäuser, & Garbade, 2015). Meta-analytic findings also suggest that self-compassion interventions of various kinds (verbal, written, training) are associated with increases in wellbeing and self-compassion (Zessin et al., 2015). A non-judgemental and compassionate attitude toward one's problems can reduce distress (MacBeth & Gumley, 2012).

One *TRANScending Love* participant described how sharing lived experiences and self-acceptance helped her feel connected: "It's really nice to share stories from people just like me, 'cause sometimes it's hard to find people that have actually been through the same thing and understand what you are going through, so you don't feel alone" (Logie et al., 2019, p. 41). This reflects the common humanity versus isolation components of self-compassion. Another participant discussed the impact of the rare opportunity to practice kindness with others: "I think the more we can celebrate our love for each other, and doing that work of self-care of saying we're beautiful to each other. That's something that I think is hard for us to do, 'cause we get the opposite messages all the time. This was really magical" (Logie et al., 2019, p. 43). Yasmeen's discussion of joyfulness, celebration, and connection in her cooking group with trans persons of colour shows the importance of fostering common humanity and self-worth, central elements of self-compassion that in turn provide hope.

4.6 Rethinking Hard to Reach Through Critical Hope

Taken together, critical hope and self-compassion approaches recognize struggles and pain, our shared humanity, and the possibility of change. Both include intrapersonal dimensions, such as values, attitudes and beliefs, and interpersonal dimensions, including our relationships and connectedness with others. Each can be applied to understanding how we can sustain work for social justice. Social justice work can also be extended to include struggles for self-acceptance and community building among stigmatized and marginalized communities, such as trans women of colour. There are differences of course between critical hope and self-compassion. Freire viewed critical hope as essential for the pursuit of social justice, while Neff conceptualizes self-compassion as key for each of us individually to live in a way that recognizes our interconnectedness. Both approaches can support social justice goals: critical hopefulness fuels us to create social transformation, while self-compassion helps us to focus on personal struggles in a way that fosters interconnectedness rather than isolation. hooks reminds us that for communities at the margins, resistance can mean imagining new futures and alternatives. For trans women of colour, social justice work is embedded in the lived experiences of navigating daily barriers of transphobia, racism and misogyny while hoping, and working, for an improved future for trans women in solidarity with others.

What then are implications of critical hopefulness and self-compassion for HIV researchers? First, as described in the reflection on *TRANScending Love* and in the conversation with Yasmeen, there is a need for researchers to move beyond a dominant focus on HIV among trans women of colour and other marginalized groups toward self-acceptance and a more holistic perspective on wellbeing. Participants articulated the importance of self-worth as a motivator to engage in HIV preventive practices. Researchers can also expand the content and foci of HIV studies to include pathways to self-acceptance and self-compassion when working with groups at the margins. A self-compassion approach can guide researchers to focus on shared suffering as part of common humanity that helps to build community and solidarity, approaching mistakes by researchers and the communities researchers work with as part of the shared human experience, and practising self-kindness. In time, this could result in research that is more meaningful and attractive to engage in for persons labelled hard to reach.

Focusing on journeys from pain to self-acceptance can also open up what hooks (1989) described as marginal spaces of possibility. One *TRANScending Love* participant recounts the importance of research activities that provide spaces for trans persons to connect:

> There's not a lot of space where trans and nonbinary people can meet, and be free, and the spaces are very limited. And, there's certain things that we can't talk about and there's certain things that we can, and I feel like we need to start creating spaces around like language, we need to start creating spaces around body image, and self-worth, what's surgery looks like, what it doesn't look like, or, self-motivation (Logie et al., 2019, p. 41).

Researchers should also consider ways to spark hope and joy in the research process. What would it look like to include critical hopefulness in our research approach, activities, and questions? Acknowledging the ways that people both struggle with social exclusion and survive and find joy, can produce more authentic and strengths-focused research. As Yasmeen described it, researchers need to expand the gaze beyond hardship: "You are going through this rough thing, but there are parts of you and things that you are doing that are amazing." Being able to hold painful experiences while creating space for new possibilities can be empowering for participants and something researchers can facilitate by ensuring that they also inquire about hopes, dreams, coping and other strengths. A *TRANScending Love* participant described how sharing her lived experiences with other trans women provided her with a fuller outlook: "When you come into a space like this, and you talk about your own personal experience, you think 'Ok, I never looked at it in this perspective'. There's a brighter, more fulfilling feeling of knowing a better way" (Logie et al., 2019, p. 42).

Researchers can also work in partnership with communities to develop research questions that elicit hope and explore the balance between challenges and strengths. Providing participants with opportunities to share hopes for social change, and to reflect on the individual and collective capacities they developed from struggle and hardship, can amplify what Freire referred to as the critical hope that already exists within us all.

Part of this shift toward hopefulness and joy is celebration. Celebration is radically understudied as a research method. We can celebrate by sharing findings in community events, using arts-based approaches that give back to participants and communities, and provide the opportunity to share food and laughter. In our work we used travelling arts exhibits, for example, printed hundreds of decks of *TRANScending Love* cards created from participants' anatomical heart drawings and affirmation cards, and held a community panel with food at a Black AIDS service organization to share *TRANScending Love* findings. Sharing this art in community spaces provided the opportunity for participants to see their work disseminated to a larger audience, and provided researchers, community members, and service providers with a glimpse into the hearts, hopes, and strengths of trans women of colour.

Turning the lens on our own growth as researchers, what would it look like if we practised self-compassion not only in research but in our own lives? Would it help us to see our common humanity with the 'hard to reach' groups we are trying to engage in our research? Would we develop more sensitive research approaches that recognize the worth, dignity, hopes, and dreams that we share with research participants? If finding space for celebration and joy in research activities can help participants to value themselves, it may also help researchers to see their interconnectedness and their shared hopes for being seen and valued.

Yasmeen called for researchers to remove their academic or research 'hats' and to connect with their souls when doing research. Critical hopefulness can amplify our ability to use research as a tool for social change, as well as stir up hope in the communities we work with to transform personal and collective futures. Yasmeen also advised researchers to remember the human aspects of research, and the practice of self-compassion can remind us of our shared humanity. Freire once called for us to challenge "coldness or indifference toward the legitimate human interests of the dispossessed—being, living with dignity, loving, studying, reading the world and the word, overcoming fear, believing, resting, dreaming, doing things, questioning, choosing, saying no at the appropriate time, cultivating a permanent yes perspective toward life" (Freire, 2004, p. 104). Critical hope and self compassion can therefore be transformative in our own lives as well as our research approaches. Both in turn will make it less likely we find that persons are hard to reach.

References

Barnett, T., Seeley, J., Levin, J., & Katongle, J. (2015). Hope: A new approach to understanding structural factors in HIV acquisition. *Global Public Health, 10*(4), 417–437.

Christens, B. D., Byrd, K., Peterson, N. A., & Lardier, D. T. (2018). Critical hopefulness among urban high school students. *Journal of Youth and Adolescence, 47*(8), 1649–1662.

Christens, B. D., Collura, J. J., & Tahir, F. (2013). Critical hopefulness: A person-centered analysis of the intersection of cognitive and emotional empowerment. *American Journal of Community Psychology, 52*(1–2), 170–184.

Ciarrochi, J., Parker, P., Kashdan, T. B., Heaven, P. C. L., & Barkus, E. (2015). Hope and emotional well-being: A six-year study to distinguish antecedents, correlates, and consequences. *The Journal of Positive Psychology, 10*(6), 520–532.

de Souza, H., & Parker, R. (1994). *The cure of AIDS*. Rio de Janeiro: Dumara.

Farran, C. J., Herth, K. A., & Popovich, J. M. (1995). *Hope and hopelessness: Critical clinical constructs*. Thousand Oaks, CA: Sage.

Freire, P. (1972). *Pedagogy of the oppressed*. London: Penguin Books.

Freire, P. (2004). *Pedagogy of indignation*. Boulder, CO: Paradigm Publishers.

Freire, P. (2007). *Daring to dream*. Boulder, CO: Paradigm Publishers.

Freire, P. (2014). *Pedagogy of hope: Reliving pedagogy of the oppressed*. New York: Bloomsbury Publishing.

Freire, P. (2016). *Pedagogy of the heart* (Bloomsbury Revelations edition). Bloomsbury Publishing, New York

Freire, P., & Macedo, D. (2003). Rethinking literacy: A dialogue. In A. Darder, M. Baltodano, & R. Torres (Eds.), *The critical pedagogy reader* (pp. 354–364). New York: RoutledgeFalmer.

Herth, K. (2000). Enhancing hope in people with a first recurrence of cancer. *Journal of Advanced Nursing, 32*(6), 1431–1441.

Herth, K. A. (2001). Development and implementation of a Hope Intervention Program. *Oncology Nursing Forum, 28*(6), 1009–1016.

hooks, b. (1989). Choosing the margin as a space of radical openness. *Framework: The Journal of Cinema and Media, 36*, 15–23.

hooks, b. (2003). *Teaching community: A pedagogy of hope*. New York: Routledge.

Logie, C. H., Lacombe-Duncan, A., Persad, Y., Ferguson, T. B., Yehdego, D. M., Ryan, S., Forrester, M., Moses, C., & Guta, A. (2019). The TRANScending love arts-based workshop to address self-acceptance and intersectional stigma among transgender women of color in Toronto, Canada: Findings from a qualitative implementation science study. *Transgender Health, 4*(1), 35–45.

MacBeth, A., & Gumley, A. (2012). Exploring compassion: A meta-analysis of the association between self-compassion and psychopathology. *Clinical Psychology Review, 32*(6), 545–552.

Miller, J. F. (2007). Hope: A construct central to nursing. *Nursing Forum, 42*(1), 12–19.

Neff, K. (2003). Self-compassion: An alternative conceptualization of a healthy attitude toward oneself. *Self and Identity, 2*(2), 85–101.

Neff, K., & Knox, M. C. (2017). Self-compassion. In V. Zeigler-Hill & T. K. Shackelford (Eds.), *Encyclopedia of personality and individual differences* (pp. 1–8). Springer International Publishing.

Snyder, C. (2000). Genesis: The birth and growth of hope. In C. Snyder (Ed.), *Handbook of hope* (pp. 25–38). San Diego, CA: Academic Press.

Snyder, C. R., Lopez, S. J., & Pedrotti, J. T. (2015). *Positive psychology: The scientific and practical explorations of human strengths* (3rd ed.). Thousand Oaks, CA: Sage.

Van Hooft, S. (2014). *Hope*. New York: Routledge.

Watney, S. (2000). *Imagine hope: AIDS and gay identity*. London: Routledge.
Webb, D. (2010). Paulo Freire and 'the need for a kind of education in hope'. *Cambridge Journal of Education, 40*(4), 327–339.
Weis, R., & Speridakos, E. C. (2011). A meta-analysis of hope enhancement strategies in clinical and community settings. *Psychology of Well-Being: Theory, Research and Practice, 1*(1), 5.
Zessin, U., Dickhäuser, O., & Garbade, S. (2015). The relationship between self-compassion and well-being: A meta-analysis. *Applied Psychology: Health and Well-Being, 7*(3), 340–364.

Chapter 5
Imagination and Possibility

This chapter describes a community-based research study developed in collaboration with *The Rock of Hope*, an LGBT community organization in Eswatini (formerly Swaziland) focused on providing LGBT advocacy and support to individuals, families, and communities. In the project, we used participatory theatre approaches to understand and address the stigma experienced by LGBT persons in Eswatini—a country in which same sex sexual practices are criminalized.

We developed three skits with *The Rock of Hope* and a theatre group. These used forum theatre techniques to engage the audience in the storytelling process. I begin by reflecting on the study, and experience developing the LGBT stigma reduction intervention in a context where same sex practices are criminalized. Next, I describe a reflective conversation with Veli Madau who worked as a research assistant on the study. Finally, I explore the wider literature on imagination and possibility as approaches to create space for researchers to work together with community members to advance social justice.

5.1 Reflections on a Participatory Theatre Project with an LGBT Community Agency, *The Rock of Hope*, in Eswatini

During the AIDS 2012 conference in Washington, D.C., a colleague and I went to a party one evening. At this party I was introduced to Xolile 'Malume' (uncle) Mabuza, a long time LGBT activist in Eswatini. Malume had an enormous laugh and huge smile and we had an animated conversation about our respective LGBT community activism. He invited me to visit *The Rock of Hope* in Eswatini, an organization he had founded many years ago before as a support group for LGBT persons. Soon after it was established, Malume was requested to talk with parents to help them accept their LGBT children, and this work later expanded to talking with

C. Logie, *Working with Excluded Populations in HIV*, Social Aspects of HIV 8,
https://doi.org/10.1007/978-3-030-77048-8_5

chiefs in rural villages to advocate for LGBT acceptance. *The Rock of Hope* grew to have its own office, hire staff, and provide LGBT social support services as well as HIV information. We planned a research study together to reduce LGBT stigma among healthcare providers and community members using participatory theatre. There were several learning moments for me during this study, including within the research process itself.

The most powerful part for me about this research project was the friendship that grew between Malume and myself. Each time I arrived in Eswatini, Malume would greet me at the airport with a radiant smile and drive me through the beautiful green hills to a restaurant overlooking a cliff. We would have a cold drink and talk about life and our research. I learned about the struggles that Malume had experienced as a trans person, leader and advocate in Eswatini. I heard stories about family and love, met his mother and son, saw the small hairdressing business he had built, and stayed at his family compound on my last research visit. The car we drove around in broke down during every single visit, causing us to spend hours talking and waiting by the side of a dusty road for someone to help to fix the tire or repair the engine. Over two and a half years of close, challenging work together culminated in a community event to share the study findings with participants and collaborators. Malume hit on the idea of using a huge piece of canvas to depict a tree, and have people paint their hands and create a tree of rainbow handprints to reflect our interconnectedness.

I had no idea that would be the last time I saw Malume. A few months after the community event I received a call from the colleague who had introduced us years before, informing me that Malume had died suddenly of a heart attack.[1] This was the first time I had lost a close friend or colleague and I was devastated. I could not focus on analysing the data or writing up the manuscripts from our study. It was in fact several years before I could analyze and present our findings, and each time I did I held back tears. I still think of Malume and the devastating loss of an LGBT activist considered an elder in the movement, only in their early fifties, in a country such as Eswatini where colonial legacies criminalizing same sex sexual practices remain. I also think of the resistance, strength, skill and creativity it took for Malume to build a national agency that still remains active years following their death to advocate for LGBT rights, and to work with families, religious and traditional leaders to change community norms to be more accepting. This experience of losing a close colleague and friend has helped me to better appreciate and nurture relationships within the research process.

There were other key moments of learning that changed my perspective on my role as a researcher. Our study involved first conducting in-depth qualitative interviews with LGBT persons in Eswatini. We analyzed these interviews together to identify scenarios to develop into skits with a local theatre group. Following the format of participatory theatre, the skits were performed in front of audiences twice: first, the skit was performed so as to culminate in a crisis, with no solution offered;

[1]https://ilga.org/14-september-2015-press-statement-immediate-release-condolence-loss-xolile-sane-mabuza.

following this, the skit was performed again, stopped at a critical juncture and an audience member invited to come up on the stage to demonstrate a solution. As the focus was on LGBT stigma, we developed three scenarios building on the study's qualitative findings and conversations with *The Rock of Hope* and the theatre group. The first skit included a young man whose mother started shouting at him to leave the house when she walked in to find him kissing with another young man. The second concerned a lesbian who went for an STI test and was told she had to bring her sex partner along for treatment, but when she brought along her girlfriend she was ridiculed by a nurse. The third scenario showed a trans women being fired by her employer after a gender transition. These skits were developed and performed to a range of participants, including community members, educators, nursing students, and healthcare providers.

There were several critical junctures at which I made the decision to enter the spaces of knowledge production to disrupt processes that reproduced LGBT stigma. These critical junctures occurred in the process of developing the skits with the theatre group, and also in the focus groups following the skits with audience members. The first of them took place when a theatre group member repeatedly misgendered Malume. Each time Malume patiently corrected them with the correct pronouns, but the member continued to refer to them with the incorrect gender. After watching this continue to happen, I decided to use my authority to interrupt. I reminded the theatre group member that the objective of participatory theatre was to reduce LGBT stigma and discrimination and to raise awareness to promote social change in Eswatini to increase the wellbeing and inclusion of LGBT persons. As we had trusted the theatre group to help us create and perform the skits, social change was also needed within the theatre group itself. I pointed to this example of continually misgendering someone after being corrected as something we need to change to reduce the stigma and exclusion directed toward trans persons in Eswatini. Directly addressing this issue was uncomfortable for me as I would have much preferred to follow the leadership of a local community group to avoid acting as a 'white saviour' or exerting my power over community leaders. I felt in this case that the disrespect and unwillingness to listen to the leader of the community partner was unacceptable and harmful, and this sparked my decision to intervene. Afterwards, Malume and I discussed this intervention and he shared it was helpful for someone else to step in to name the stigma when their own voice was being ignored.

Two other occasions on which I disrupted stigma and discrimination occurred during the participatory theatre workshops themselves. On the first day when we divided the audience participants into smaller focus groups following the performance, one participant repeatedly told the other focus group participants that LGBT people were sinners and would go to hell. Occasionally, in past studies I have interrupted or corrected focus group participants when they shared misinformation or were offensive to other participants. I stepped in and informed this participant that their beliefs were stigmatizing and this was not an appropriate place to display such condemning attitudes. He would not stop, however, so I met with the community partners and told them that we needed to ask him to leave as he was being disruptive. As they did not want to damage their relationships with the individual, they asked me to tell him to leave. I felt uncomfortable about this but knew that the longer he stayed in the focus group sharing these beliefs, the greater the likelihood that he would offend the LGBT persons in the room and the less time there would be for other focus group participants to share their experiences. While he agreed to leave, he returned the following day for the second participatory theatre event. Our community partners in Eswatini again did not feel comfortable asking him to leave, so again I had to ask him to do. This was hard to do as a young, white, foreign, queer woman but it was also necessary to avoid the disruption that would result from having an openly stigmatizing and disruptive participant.

A third example of interrupting stigma happened during the skit about the trans woman who lost her employment after her gender transition. When we asked a participant in the audience to step into the role of the employer to re-enact a more supportive response than her firing, the participant responded by informing the trans woman that she could keep her employment but only if she worked at the back of the shop where none of the customers could see her. While technically this might be considered preferable to firing an employee, I did not feel comfortable leaving the audience thinking that this was an acceptable solution. I therefore asked *The Rock of Hope* if one of their members could act out an even more supportive response, specifically requesting them play the role of an employer who welcomed the employee back and let them keep the same job interacting with customers. We then enacted the skit a third time modelling this supportive employer response. Afterwards, I reflected on the situation and considered the challenges in a context such as Eswatini, where same sex practices remain criminalized and there are no LGBT human rights protections, for a member of the general public to imagine what a supportive and gender affirming response might look like in the workplace. Expecting heterosexual, cisgender people who are not familiar with LGBT issues to role model a supportive response might—but might not—produce the results we are hoping for. I also thought about Malume, and the vision of new possibilities they had had when starting a LGBT support group from their home and growing it into national platform, maintaining a steadfast belief in the possibility of communities, families and leaders changing to become the supportive allies of LGBT persons.

5.2 In Conversation: Veli Madau

Carmen: *I am happy to be talking with you about our project with The Rock of Hope. What was your experience overall like with this project?*

Veli: *What I remember from the project was getting a chance to hear people's stories and from those stories, what was interesting is being able to recognize the common themes that came across different individuals. At that time, we had not had any formal research for LGBTI (lesbian, gay, bisexual, transgender and intersex) people in Swaziland. It was an interesting project. That was the first to actually capture data in a way that we actually published papers out of it, as well as the recognition of the similarities that we have as LGBTI people in that space.*

It also was recognizing how often we do not get an opportunity to talk about that, especially being able to share those experiences with people who identify as LGBTI. Sharing these experiences in the skits allowed for a good conversation starter. It is hard to just come across a person and tell them your life story and all of your experiences. But when people saw in the skits what LGBTI people experienced, somehow it made them relate a little bit more with us.

Carmen: *Can we go back a little? I am curious how you became involved with Rock of Hope.*

Veli: *My involvement with The Rock of Hope began when I had time on my hands and found this organization for LGBTI people in Swaziland. I volunteered and offered my IT (information technology) services. That is how I started getting involved with this research project and realized that there is an opportunity to actually make a difference in Swaziland. After Malume passed away, I had to take on a lot of responsibility in the organization until a time came where I just could not balance that and my work. It is a struggle to fund LGBTI organizing, so it is difficult for people to actually make a living out of activism.*

Carmen: *What is your relationship like with The Rock of Hope or other LGBTI agencies today?*

Veli: *I do still do advocacy with an informal queer women's collective. We got together with the understanding that a lot of the organizations that are in existence are primarily pushing gay men, and other men who have sex with men, mandates due to where the HIV funding is coming from. We felt we needed to look for opportunities to specifically explore issues that lesbian, bisexual and trans women face.*

Carmen: *That is amazing. I have been thinking about the idea that LGBTI people could be considered hard to reach in Swaziland. What was your experience like doing interviews for this research project?*

Veli: *It was not that LGBTI people were particularly hard to find at the time. When interviewing people and approaching people, it was mostly people I did not know. And that, for me, was interesting. I did not have any preconceptions about people while interviewing. I do know that in the team we had some people who were involved within the community for some time before the project started. I think it influenced participation and also the honesty in which people were sharing their stories. If someone knew someone from before, you would find that a person may not have been willing to share as much of their story as they would have if it was someone they did not know. I did not feel that with people that I had to interview. Except the one interview where the person was familiar to me was the most uncomfortable. I think they wanted to portray themselves in a particular way. Opening up and showing vulnerabilities was not as easy.*

Carmen: *That is very true. When you were looking for people to participate, why were they willing to come?*

Veli: *Participation was because The Rock of Hope was doing a lot of work and very visible in the country. When you heard "The Rock of Hope" people wanted to participate. Also, there was this organization to connect with for those who had not heard about it. We were trying to reach more people, to move beyond the circle of* *people that might already come into The Rock of Hope. It is important to include more voices, as there are experiences that would hold true for a certain group of people, but not so true for others.*

Carmen: *I wanted to ask you about something that happened in the research process that I found challenging. The theatre group we worked with kept misgendering persons, and I had to keep correcting them. What has your experience been with addressing (or not addressing) misgendering?*

Veli: *It is very, very common, particularly for people like my myself. I present in a very masculine way, but I identify as female. When I first started working, you would find people referring to me as 'he' and people getting uncomfortable with the pronouns. There are some organizations that have open and allow safe spaces for people to ask you what your pronouns are and allow for that kind of conversation.*

But there are spaces where there is a lot of misgendering. And there is a misconception where people still think that lesbians are just trying to be to be men. Therefore, people would want to address them using male pronouns. And it is very, very, very common to have that. Sometimes people intentionally do that, even when they can see that you are you are female. It is not usually done in a pleasant way of recognizing or trying to understand your sexuality.

Carmen: *So that is something that is common. When do you know when to say something and not to say something? How do you navigate that?*

Veli: *It is not all the time that you would make a correction. It has become intuitive more than certain, and it is based on knowing yourself and your surroundings. When I started working for the first few months, I was not as comfortable to speak about my sexuality with everyone because I was not sure about the environment. But as soon as I realized the type of environment and who I was in that space, the organization and the culture, I found that I was basically protected by the space. I was able to have open conversations, but also the type of people who are in this space are open minded enough to have those conversations. It is different when you are in, for example, government places where you will get reluctance and discrimination if you were to say anything. In government places if someone were to address me as a man, I would not make that correction because of the repercussions of me telling them that I am a woman in that space and I am wearing pants. I think it comes with knowing your surroundings and knowing when to speak your voice and also, for issues of safety, sometimes you would not want to make that correction.*

I am very open to making that that correction when accessing public toilets. You would not want to use the male toilets. You will make that correction to say you are using the women's toilets because you are a female. And it is interesting because this is the toilet that you are supposed to be using. For me, it is an issue of safety and the surrounding.

Carmen: *You are so right, and this issue of gender policing in bathrooms is so global. I remember you and others did amazing work with the chiefs around gender norms in clothing.*

Veli: *In cultural spaces or events where you are expected to wear traditional clothes, in family events or work events, I intentionally wear what customarily would be worn by men. I do get stares. For me, in just my existence and my living, I would* *like to show people that we should be allowed to express ourselves, regardless of how society is trying to shape us or dictate how we should live our lives or how we should express ourselves. By just waking up and going to the office, I have realized that just my existence is opening people's minds to learning about or to be curious enough to ask questions about LGBTI people. In the health care sector now, I have had conversations with people who I have worked with when I was an activist at The Rock of Hope but did not have the opportunity to connect with. Now being in a space where we are all professionals and focused on HIV, they are relating with me from that perspective as opposed to seeing me as somebody who is totally different. So now we are talking about sexuality like any other conversation, such as "how are you and what did you eat in the morning?" It becomes a normal part of a conversation as opposed to something that is so totally out of place in that space.*

Carmen: *That is a major shift, from the LGBTI agency as an activist to an HIV research agency.*

Veli: *I have recognized that it has become easier to interact with people. I am not coming in as an advocate, but I am coming in as a colleague. As a colleague we are relating first on the issues that we need to talk about, on our health care's perspective on HIV. But also, I am an LGBTI identifying individual and I am part of this community. I have had people ask personal questions and really ask "what does that mean for you?" Those kinds of questions that are not derogatory, but questions where people are curious to know, to understand, and not just to tick a box. It is different when people see you as a person first and then they are able to have a conversation with you as opposed to someone seeing you as something that is different. You already have so much work to do to just be seen as a person before you can even start talking about who you are and your experiences in life. I think being in a certain space allows people to see you differently.*

Carmen: *That is so powerful. Do you remember we did three theater skits: one had a transgender woman who had recently transitioned who came back to work and was fired. What was a learning moment for me was when we froze that skit, and someone came in from the audience and their solution as the employer was to tell the trans woman actor, "I'm not going to fire you, but you have to work in the back so that no one can see you." I remember feeling alarmed as that was not the message I wanted all of the participants to leave with. So, I asked someone from The Rock of Hope to go in and do the skit a third time to act in a more supportive way to get the message across. I thought maybe it was too hard to model behavior that no one has seen before. Maybe nobody actually knows the ideal way of treating a trans person. I wonder what you thought about that.*

Veli: *I think one of the learnings I got from that was I do not think there is one answer or one solution. You can get a different number of ways in which you can have an ending from someone in the audience. There is a way which people should not be treating LGBTI people. The message that should come is to treat a person in a way that you would also want to be treated. When you are put in a position that makes you uncomfortable, it helps you to think about how you treat another person in that situation. Making it personal so people understand that this could happen to anybody at any time.*

Look, this is not even particularly about sexuality, but humanizing those scenarios in such a way that the take home message is how you feel. To create the message that yes, we are treating a human being at the end of the day. Whatever you do should be something that you would also want to be treated like. Teaching people to reflect on how they want to be treated—to put yourself in that person's shoes. We need to focus on the emotion more than the action. The actions are actually coming from how you are feeling at the time.

Carmen: *A lot of what I'm writing about in this book is about reflecting on ourselves, and considering how we can use love and care to guide our research. If someone was going to do research right now with LGBTI people in Swaziland, what is important to know?*

Veli: *To tell the story of an LGBTI person requires an LGBTI person to tell that story. But getting that story to be received is different: you need to think how you can get someone else to be interested enough to want to hear that story. And not just to hear it, but to do something about it. Telling your story and opening up your vulnerabilities without knowing how you will be received is difficult. And once you have opened yourself up, you cannot go back. I think the best outcome is if the story can be told directly by the person. But it is difficult to get that story direct from a person for issues of safety, and also not knowing how you would be received. So often people end up having to have someone else narrate the story because of the audience. What happens often is there is an LGBTI community group, they are doing the research with LGBTI persons but do not have a formal methodology. For researchers, that data is invalid. Yet those stories are so true to the people telling those stories. They are invalid because the community groups were not aware of the audience that they wanted to share those stories with. The stories are there and we know the best thing is to get the stories from the people. But how can these those stories be delivered to different audiences in ways that the message is best received?*

Carmen: *That is such good advice. What you are saying is there is a lot of data, a lot of stories, that have been collected but because it was done in informal ways by LGBTI community groups it is hard to get this data recognized.*

Veli: *Yes, I think the mood within the LGBTI community is that for some time a lot of people in LGBTI organizations or as part of the movement have not had opportunities; they have been turned back from other spaces of employment or even basic educational settings. They have found a home in the LGBTI movement. Therefore, what we call research in the LGBTI movement versus what we term research in academic institutions is different. In having conversations with people from the LGBTI community, people felt that people would come with degrees and come with very good proposals and get data from the community. It was very extractive as the people who are sharing their stories and giving the data do not get anything out of that. That has created a bit of reluctance from people in the LGBTI community to be open and share their stories.*

Carmen: *What do you think would be the ideal way that an academic researcher would work with the LGBTI community in Swaziland?*

Veli: *I have thought about this for quite some time. I do not have a straightforward or short answer, but what I know is there needs to be a different way by which* *we share the findings. If we are writing an academic paper, it excludes a lot of the people who are in the LGBTI community. If you are in the community doing your own research, you cannot publish that paper in a journal. So, I do not know if there is a way in disseminating your results that can also be appreciated by the community.*

Carmen: *I think that is such a good point so the community can get the findings in a way that they can understand. We had a community forum where we shared the findings with a lot of stakeholders and that included an art project with participants. We also could have shared the findings in different ways, such as a postcard or comic. For me, this was a very hard project to finish after Malume died. It took me 2 years to even be able to look at the data. It was such a hard loss.*

Veli: *It was heartbreaking. For the community, I think for us losing somebody who had dedicated so much to the movement, really hit us all hard. For us to actually get something out of the data... we pushed to not let all of that work be done in vain. Let us see what we can get out of that. Part of why I sacrificed so much after Malume passed away, balancing pressure from work while trying to manage The Rock of Hope, was to try and keep it afloat to let all of that work serve some purpose.*

Carmen: *This book is dedicated to Malume. I learned so much from them about joy. This person sacrificed so much to build the LGBT community, starting The Rock of Hope from their house and growing it into a national agency. Overcoming barriers, including having their house burnt down, and being arrested. Malume had so much hardship and was always so positive and hopeful. Willing to give so much to others, travelling all over Swaziland to connect with chiefs, parents, LGBTI persons, willing to help anybody. I have never met anybody like that.*

Veli: *He really touched a lot of lives. Even now when we are talking about the work that we are doing, we still make reference to a lot of valuable lessons that we learned from Malume. Embracing life and all of its difficulties and approaching it all with love and joy really makes a difference in what you do. Hardships will always be there, but all in all, your attitude towards it makes a difference in how you to continue living.*

Carmen: *What does it mean to be loving in your research? I have been thinking about hospitality. Every single time I came to Swaziland Malume picked me up from the airport and took me to this restaurant overlooking the mountains and we would have a drink. It was just this feeling of being cared for.*

Veli: *Still to this day I think of how it takes a lot of strength and maturity to understand how, in spite of all the things that happened to you and all the things that are happening, you can still choose to be happy, to be joyful, and to push forward love. One of the great lessons I learnt from Malume was that of love and keeping a cheerful spirit. His joyful and welcoming nature attracted so much for the organization and also for the country. We are still getting organizations and people that just want to be involved in LGBTI work in Swaziland because of Malume.*

Carmen: *To think that you could really forgive and keep going forward because your vision was way bigger than yourself. They were doing this to help younger people, to help families.*

Veli: *One thing that Malume would always say is that with all the things that they were doing, it was not for them. It was with the understanding that there is a generation that is coming after and they should find things in a better space than they were before. I think they did a good job with that. And I live my life with the acknowledgment that my existence and presentation daily is a form of passive activism, and I believe we can all make a difference in our different spaces, every contribution is invaluable.*

5.3 Applying Concepts of Imagination and Possibility to Work with Socially Excluded Populations

> Marginality is much more than a site of deprivation, in fact... it is also the site of radical possibility, a space of resistance. It was this marginality that I was naming as a central location for the production of a counter-hegemonic discourse that is not just found in words but in habits of being and the way one lives (hooks, 1984, p. 203).

As hooks (1984) describes above, research with people who are marginalized can move beyond centering oppression to examine resistance and spaces of possibility for social change. Theatre and performance have been used to generate such opportunities for change since the early days of the epidemic. For instance, *Theatre Rhinoceros* (1977–2001) was a gay and lesbian theatre company in San Francisco founded by Allan Estes who died of AIDS-related complications in 1984. Through its work, it reflected the gay and lesbian liberation "movement's coming of age. No longer hiding in, or hidden by a heterosexual theatre world, these gay-oriented artists actively explored the dimensions of their own sexuality and the dynamics of same-sex relationships in an environment ostensibly free from the hegemony of traditional, heterosexual, 'mainstream' theatre" (MacDonald, 1989, p. 79). Estes founded the gay and lesbian theatre company to enrich the lives of both artists and audience members, and topics addressed included gay persons' experiences with coming out, sexual intimacy between men, violent victimization (such as 'gay bashing'), HIV and AIDS, and resistance to oppression and violence (MacDonald, 1989). Their production "*Artists Involved with Death and Survival: The A.I.D.S. Show*" depicted the early days of the pandemic through scenarios from New Year's Eve parties spanning 1980 to 1984. These depicted caring for people living with HIV, a mother accepting her gay son, and persons engaging with safer sex practices. In this way, the *A.I.D.S. Show* moved beyond suffering and death to offer an empowering perspective on gay and lesbian experiences. Celebration of life and freedom of gay and lesbian communities and their "irrepressible will to be free" (MacDonald, 1989, p. 92) in the context of stigma, discrimination, and the HIV epidemic was a central tenet of *Theatre Rhinoceros*. This suggests theatre can be a place in which perspectives toward marginalized communities and issues may be changed. Radical imagination and possibility may be helpful concepts for researchers working with socially excluded persons, such as LGBT persons in contexts where same sex practices are criminalized.

5.3.1 Participatory Theatre and Vernacular Knowledge

> In its most essential sense, theatre is the capacity possessed by human beings—and not by animals—to observe themselves in action. Humans are capable of seeing themselves in the act of seeing, of thinking their emotions, of being moved by their thoughts. They can see themselves here and imagine themselves there; they can see themselves today and imagine themselves tomorrow (Boal & Jackson, 2005, p. 11).

Power shapes the dynamic production and recognition of knowledge. Language can reproduce dominant power systems, including through its devaluation of vernacular language (hooks, 1989). Vernacular—or 'everyday'—knowledge includes local, community situated knowledge and its interaction with formal knowledge and 'expertise', largely controlled by political and scientific institutions. Escoffier (1998) has described how:

> Vernacular knowledge is dispersed throughout society; it is a component in everyday social interactions, skills, practices, social networks, and institutions. . .Every social actor possesses a stock of vernacular knowledge that is assembled from the everyday 'learning by doing', the responses to challenges, and personal observation (p. 4).

Vernacular knowledge comprises the larger belief systems that generate meaning and identity, shape practices, and build solidarity between social groups. In essence, vernacular knowledge shapes the way we live our everyday lives—including gender roles and expectations, biases and stereotypes, and social hierarchies. Vernacular knowledge challenges authoritative knowledge structures, yet it is systematically marginalized by scientific and political knowledge production (Escoffier, 1998). In our reflective conversation above, Veli discussed how the knowledge generated by LGBT community members about their own lived experiences is often overlooked by researchers. This results in research projects—including our own study—not sharing results back in ways that resonate with the vernacular knowledge of local LGBT persons.

There is a long history of vernacular knowledge being leveraged for HIV prevention, including in safer sex campaigns with gay and bisexual men (Escoffier, 1998; Martos, 2016). In HIV advocacy, outreach, and prevention, different actors (epidemiology, gay communities) compete for knowledge and power. On the one hand, gay communities may seek to resist stigma and pathologizing discourses, aiming to build on community strengths and lived experiences in prevention efforts. On the other hand, public health, political and religious actors may focus on identifying 'high risk' groups and advocate for social controls—including targeting the 'homosexual lifestyle'—through punitive measures such as closing down bathhouses. The pamphlet *How to Have Sex in an Epidemic* was developed by Richard Berkowitz, Michael Callen and Richard Dworkin, with scientific and medical input from Joseph Sonnabend, very early in the epidemic in 1983 in New York City as a means for gay communities to harness community practices of care, love, and intimacy (rather than fear of infection) to increase the uptake of HIV prevention practices (Berkowitz, Callen, & Dworkin, 1983). Yet the allocation of resources based on who is constructed as at risk for HIV in contexts such as Eswatini where there exist no LGBT human rights protections overlooks lesbian and bisexual women who can benefit from LGBT community, sexual rights advocacy and solidarity building (Logie, 2014; Logie & Gibson, 2013). Veli identified how dominant HIV risk categorizations have shaped the exclusion of lesbian and bisexual women from HIV funding in Eswatini, sparking her own involvement in a movement focused on "issues that lesbian, bisexual and trans women face in particular".

Challenging stigma therefore includes critically examining how knowledge is organized and produced while amplifying vernacular knowledge as a means to engage community knowledge in problem solving. Freire's pedagogy of the oppressed focused on the humanization and liberation of marginalized persons through education (Freire, 1972). The process of liberation results in persons being able to live their lives authentically by controlling their own pedagogy in ways that foster open questioning, critical thinking, and recognition of where and how their humanity is being limited. Freire's approach aligns with Escoffier's wish to harness vernacular knowledge within social excluded communities to generate solidarity and support people to live authentically and realize their humanity (Martos, 2016). Together, these perspectives signal the importance of marginalized communities producing education and social change from below through actions rooted in vernacular knowledge. The research study discussed in this chapter aimed to identify, share, and generate vernacular knowledge using participatory theatre to generate community problem solving around the 'wicked problem' of LGBT stigma.

Language sets limits and possibilities for resistance, but these limits signal other ways of communicating to amplify multiple voices and stories—such as through theatre. Boal has described how theatre can be used as a weapon—for domination or for liberation and social change (Boal, 2014). He described how "theatre can be placed in service of the oppressed" (Boal, 2014, p. 121) by transforming passive spectators into actors with the ability to generate solutions and plans for change. Although not necessarily always revolutionary, this approach prepares the spect-actor for planning and action. Boal described the *Theatre of the Oppressed* as an approach that conceptualizes persons as both actors and spectators—*spect-actors*—who act and observe. As a critical pedagogical tool, Boal used theatre to engage with marginalized persons, first in Brazil then in global contexts, to increase critical consciousness in the form of awareness of one's social position in relationship to power and oppression (Boal, 2014). Boal expanded his theatre approach to include the wider community, including those who held more power and could be considered 'oppressors' alongside persons who were marginalized in order to spark dialogue with the goal of social change.

Forum, or participatory, theatre depicts a social or political problem with no solution being provided. In the theatre example described earlier we generated scenarios from qualitative data collected from LGBT persons in Eswatini. The audience (spect-actors) were invited to go onstage and participate in another rendition of the scenario, conducted in an identical way to the first time, in order to generate community-grounded ideas and responses. In this way, the participant/spect-actor has the opportunity to imagine and practice new ways of being and acting. Boal was clear that the spect-actor practices their ideas and solutions on stage, and that the solution is enacted and not simply discussed as it might be when sitting down on a chair. The purpose of forum theatre is not to impose ideas or solutions, but to generate a space in which people can practice possibilities and new pathways (Boal, 2014). This practising may be a rehearsal that sparks the wish to practice these new ways of being more generally. As Boal (2014) described it:

> 'Spectator' is a bad word! The spectator is less than a man and it is necessary to humanize him, to restore to him his capacity for action in all its fullness. . .all these experiments of a people's theatre have the same objective—the liberation of the spectator, on whom the theatre has imposed finished visions of the world. . .The poetics of the oppressed is essentially the poetics of liberation: the spectator no longer delegates power to the characters either to think or to act in his place. The spectator frees himself; he thinks and acts for himself! Theater is action! Perhaps the theatre is not revolutionary in itself; but have no doubts, it is a rehearsal of revolution! (p. 155).

Forum theatre has been widely used in North America to tackle LGBT stigma and in Sub-Saharan Africa to address HIV-related stigma. This chapter has looked at how we used participatory theatre as a tool to produce new awareness, foster empathy, and reduce stigmatizing attitudes and practices toward LGBT persons in Eswatini. We leveraged Boal's approach to include the targets of stigma (LGBT persons) alongside heterosexual and cisgender persons who represented the dominant social groups. Both could be considered hard to reach in contexts where same-sex practices are criminalized and there are no LGBT human rights protections. LGBT persons experience research participation barriers and may be fearful to disclose their sexual and/or gender identities, and members of the 'general public' and healthcare providers may be hard to engage in LGBT stigma reduction interventions due to fear of potential repercussions from being associated with LGBT persons. For instance, persons may fear being considered LGBT themselves, or may be punished for supporting LGBT persons. Indeed, one collaborator from Eswatini based at a Christian academic institution was reprimanded for engaging with our study because of its LGBT focus. Thus, stigmatizing contexts can make it difficult for both the targets and perpetrators of stigma to participate in social justice oriented research and in other actions to change the world, due to fear of socio-political repercussions.

When a group such as LGBT persons in Eswatini is socially and politically marginalized, researchers may find it hard to reach. Key to our reaching LGBT persons in this study was a community-based approach that foregrounded engagement with local LGBT and theatre groups in study development and implementation. LGBT community agencies and collaborators facilitated data collection from a range of participants across sexual and gender identities. The theatre group allowed the experiences of LGBT persons to be shared with the public in a safe way. Because narratives were shared by professional actors there was no need for LGBT persons to publicly disclose their identity and experience harm. We created vignettes that reflected collective, rather than individual, experiences to maintain the privacy of study participants. As the theatre group was not LGBT identified (although individual actors may have been) participants in the study could explain that they were watching a theatre performance without automatically being associated with LGBT issues. The theatre group created songs accompanied by drumming and dancing, signalling the performance was attuned to local tradition and cultural norms. Together, these considerations helped create a space in which participants felt free to engage with forum theatre and the LGBT study focus. By providing an opportunity for the "liberation of the spectator" (Boal, 2014), where participants could change the dramatic direction by generating and practising solutions, participants were actively engaged in imagining and trying out supportive, non-stigmatizing possibilities for relating with LGBT persons. They were also liberated to participate in an LGBT-focused event because of its framing as a theatre performance. For instance, one of the participatory theatre participants in our study described how:

> I feel like the way you are bringing the sensitization through the performances is louder, clearer, and it is better than having to sit through a power point presentation. It changes your attitude even better than having to buy a book, because even if there was a book about it, I do not think I would even buy it. But the performance makes me more interested, I even want to take the initiative to make this known to my institution (Logie et al., 2019).

This quotation reflects Boal's description of the theatre of the oppressed as a form of communication that can inspire real action—the participant above described how they would not have read a book on LGBT issues, yet the language of theatre moved them in such a way they were inspired to take action to bring about change in their own workplace.

Boal described "theatrical language is the most essential human language. Everything that actors do on stage, we do throughout our lives, always and everywhere" (Boal, 2002, p. 15). Theatre has the power to provoke our imagination through observing actions that spark new emotions and thoughts, and inviting us to recognize ourselves in another person or situation. As another participant in the participatory theatre event in Manzini, Eswatini described it,

> I felt happy that finally someone is actually trying to draw a real picture of what actually happens because all along I have had people talk about the situation, and trying to describe them and not actually trying to portray the real case scenario... Because sometimes you might describe and explain to people and people won't see, but through action drama that we have seen out there it actually shows in reality what is going on out there.

Participant narratives also aligned with Veli's reflection earlier in this chapter, when she highlighted the need to find creative approaches to amplify the voices of LGBT persons, while at the same time having the story received in a way that sparks social change. Our experience with participatory theatre suggests it can be a way of both sharing LGBT narratives to reduce stigma, as well as inspiring new ways of thinking and acting toward LGBT persons.

In this way, participatory theatre research creates a new opportunity for participants to learn in a visceral way about LGBT stigma, beyond what they may have understood from reading or talking about issues. It also generates empathy. As Veli described in our reflective conversation, participatory theatre taught "people to reflect on how they want to be treated—to put yourself in that person's shoes, we need to focus on the emotion more than the action." Participants discussed feeling surprised and hurt when they watched the skits and learned about the oppression and suffering LGBT people experienced, this understanding of shared humanity ignited their desire to act differently (Logie et al., 2019).

Participatory theatre's use as a research approach for creating social change signals its potential to engage multiple stakeholders in social justice-oriented projects across diverse global contexts. For instance, when LGBT youth used participatory theatre and dialogue to teach their classmates and teachers about their experiences of LGBT stigma in a study in the USA, both classmates and adult powerholders were more likely to report allyship practices, including the intention to intervene during a bullying situation (Wernick, Dessel, Kulick, & Graham, 2013), and to enact individual and institutional change (Wernick, Woodford, & Kulick, 2014).

While such a strategy has the potential to nurture empathy and inspire new perspectives and considerations for action, by itself it may not lead to long-term, durable change (Michalak et al., 2014). It therefore needs to be embedded in larger social change efforts to promote structural and systemic transformation. Some programs, such as the Young Citizens Program, have leveraged theatre as part of a larger structural approach to building self-efficacy and collective agency among young people by increasing their ability to engage in public dialogue to effect social change (Carlson, Brennan, & Earls, 2012). Participatory theatre holds promise in engaging persons with different access to power in research, providing a platform on which to amplify marginalized voices and issues in a way that engages both marginalized and more privileged communities in dialogue and solution-building for social change.

5.3.2 Broadening the Methodological Imagination

Participatory theatre can also expand our imagination. Fine discusses the importance of doing so in a way that "resituates lives in history, oppression, context" (Fine, 2007, p. 460). She pushes researchers to consider embracing ways of producing knowledge that are humanizing, rooted in socio-historic context, and which unravel the complexity within human thoughts, practices and actions. *Methodological release points* have been conceptualized by McClelland and Fine (2008) as novel research methods that create openings to disrupt what is taken for granted. They may include guided visualization, working with participants to *re-story* data, comics and graphic medicine, and other participatory action research approaches, such as the participatory theatre method we used in our study (Fine, 2007). Through the use of such techniques, research participants and researchers alike are invited to think in new ways, to imagine, and to generate novel insights contributing to social change.

The production and dissemination of insight and knowledge has material consequences, especially when translated into new skills. For instance, Fine and McClelland (2006) have signalled the importance for researchers to *thicken* theories of young women's sexual desire to move beyond a focus on victimization. When women's sexual pleasure is erased from sex education, they are not provided the knowledge and skills to negotiate pleasurable and safer sexual practices. Similarly, when LGBT persons are excluded from media, health, religious, and education systems, there will be knowledge gaps about their lived realities, experiences and needs. These absences may be considered a form of structural violence as they limit the possibilities of sexual and gender expression among all persons in a society. Social, political and health policies that constrain sexual rights and possibilities can result from this limited understanding of richness and complexity within communities.

In contrast, a *thick desire* framework can integrate socio-environmental considerations into understandings of sexuality (Fine & McClelland, 2006), including the freedom to realize sexual rights and freedom from violence that spark new imaginings for future ways of living (McClelland & Fine, 2008). Fine and McClelland describe how: "thick desire places sexual activity for all people, regardless of age or gender, within a larger context of social and interpersonal structures that enable a person to engage in the political act of wanting" (Fine & McClelland, 2006, p. 325). From this perspective, *desire* permeates minds, souls and bodies and encompasses social, economic, health and sexual factors, and *wanting* includes hopes, dreams and opportunities for the future. Such a conceptualization posits how thick desire can be both an outcome of enabling social, political and economic conditions, as well as a tool to advocate and create social change to realize such supportive environments and opportunities.

As LGBT persons in Eswatini may be framed as stigmatized victims of violence requiring human rights protection, there may be analogous benefits of considering *thick desire* in this context where the HIV prevalence of 27% among adults aged 15 to 49 is among the highest in the world (UNAIDS, 2019). For instance, the participatory theatre vignettes began with a young man kissing another man, and a young woman bringing in a same gender sex partner for STI testing. While responses to these examples of intimacy in family and healthcare settings included abuse and mistreatment, we created openings to show this intimacy in a context where most participants reported never having met an LGBT person. While we wanted to use participatory theatre as a tool to reduce stigmatizing practices and promote sexual rights for LGBT persons, our ability to create the vignettes for, and conduct, the participatory theatre project was the outcome of decades of sexual rights advocacy led by community collaborators at *The Rock of Hope*. LGBT groups in Eswatini set the stage for this work by first imagining the new possibilities of living that centered dignity, mutual support, and a society in which they would realize acceptance and rights. As McClelland and Fine describe it: "thick desire, then, may be a catalyst as well as an outcome of sexual rights" (McClelland & Fine, 2008, p. 245).

Performative methods are an approach congruent with exposing new insights and connections inspired by this focus on thick desire in ways that reflect *dramatic knowing*. The ability to experience and experiment in theatre in ways that critique the social world and imagine new possibilities aligns with Boal's description of the theatre of the oppressed. Queering the gaze to flip the viewed/viewer parallel's

Boal's discussion of the spect-actor. By facilitating a participatory theatre event with an LGBT community group for members of the general public—most whom asserted they had never met an LGBT person before—we created an opening for people to hear new stories, practice new ways of interacting with LGBT persons that disrupt stigma, and in turn unpack their own stereotypes. In this way, the project served as a *methodological release point* that contested what people thought they knew about LGBT persons in Eswatini and engaged them in imagining new ways of seeing and being in relation to the 'other.'

5.4 Rethinking Hard to Reach Through Imagination and Possibility

This chapter has explored how concepts of imagination and possibility can inform the research process, methods and outcomes. The case example described here offered the potential of using participatory theatre to engage a range of community members in generating possible ways of reducing LGBT stigma in a context where same sex sexual practices are criminalized. Research methods, such as Boal's theatre of the oppressed, can produce opportunities to imagine and practice new ways of being in the world. Participatory theatre can also amplify the presence and power of vernacular knowledge that is often overlooked in scientific research. Expanding our imagination as researchers can also include stretching the boundaries of our conversations to better understand thick desire and the ways in which people's wanting and opportunities are shaped by larger social, structural, political and economic environments.

In this study, we intentionally focused on social and structural norms and practices that shape the daily lives of LGBT persons in Eswatini. To do this, we applied a social ecological framework to reveal the multiple factors that shape and reproduce stigma: families, healthcare workers, and employers. This shifted the focus from the problem of stigma as residing in individual attitudes to one that focused the need for change on multiple facets of the social world. We also showed LGBT people as living full lives—dating, kissing, working—in criminalizing contexts, which can in itself be considered resistance. As Veli put it in our reflective conversation: "in just my existence and my living, I would like to show people that we should be allowed to express ourselves." Using LGBT narratives to situate the problem of stigma and corresponding solutions in a wider context foregrounds the need to change socio-political contexts. It also moves towards what Fine (2007) describes as *theorizing the outlier.* Rather than perceiving LGBT persons as occupying the outer margins of society (and thereby being hard to reach), we instead centered them as holders of counterhegemonic knowledge, experts on social inequity, with silenced stories of resistance and subversion. In this way, "persons presumed to be outliers" can "be theoretically reclaimed" in research (Fine, 2007, p. 469).

Researchers navigate differences in vulnerability and perspectives with communities. Being open to the unpredictability of qualitative research is a vulnerable space for researchers to operate in. Exclusions and absences may vary by type of research, but regardless, researchers can remain open to new insights, possibilities and change. In sum, the methodological imagination reminds us that research is inherently relational and that our subjectivities—including our emotions, feelings, hopes, dreams and even our bodies—are intimately entwined within it. Recognizing this can help us to consider how we react to surprises and challenges encountered in the course of research and what we can learn about ourselves in the process. To use research to spark social change, we can design studies that create opportunities for people to imagine and practice new ways of being in a more equitable world. In this chapter, our collaborator *The Rock of Hope* offered a roadmap on how to act with the intention of doing so. Veli describes this as a guiding force in Malume's work: "One thing that Malume would always say is that with all the things that they were doing, it was not for them. It was with the understanding that there is a generation that is coming after and they should find things in a better space than they were before." Research designs that create openings for imagining new possibilities can be welcoming for persons who are categorized as hard to reach.

References

Berkowitz, R., Callen, M., & Dworkin, R. (1983). *How to have sex in an epidemic: One Approach*. New York, USA: News From The Front Publications.

Boal, A. (2002). *Games for actors and non-actors*. London, UK: Routledge.

Boal, A. (2014). *Theatre of the oppressed*. New York, USA: Theatre Communications Group.

Boal, A., & Jackson, A. (2005). *Games for actors and non-actors*. London, UK: Taylor & Francis.

Carlson, M., Brennan, R. T., & Earls, F. (2012). Enhancing adolescent self-efficacy and collective efficacy through public engagement around HIV/AIDS competence: A multilevel, cluster randomized-controlled trial. *Social Science & Medicine, 75*(6), 1078–1087.

Escoffier, J. (1998). The invention of safer sex: Vernacular knowledge, Gay Politics and HIV Prevention. *Berkeley Journal of Sociology, 43*, 1–30.

Fine, M. (2007). Expanding the methodological imagination. *The Counseling Psychologist, 35*(3), 459–473.

Fine, M., & McClelland, S. (2006). Sexuality education and desire: Still missing after all these years. *Harvard Educational Review, 76*(3), 297–338.

Freire, P. (1972). *Pedagogy of the oppressed*. London, UK: Penguin Books.

hooks, b. (1984). *Feminist theory from margin to center*. Cambridge, USA: South End Press.

hooks, b. (1989). Choosing the margin as a space of radical openness. *Framework: The Journal of Cinema and Media, 36*, 15–23.

Logie, C. (2014). (Where) do queer women belong? Theorizing intersectional and compulsory heterosexism in HIV research. *Critical Public Health, 25*(5), 527–538.

Logie, C., Dias, L. V., Jenkinson, J., Newman, P. A., MacKenzie, R. K., Mothopeng, T., Madau, V., Ranotsi, A., Nhlengethwa, W., & Baral, S. D. (2019). Exploring the potential of participatory theatre to reduce stigma and promote health equity for lesbian, gay, bisexual, and transgender (LGBT) people in Swaziland and Lesotho. *Health Education & Behavior: The Official Publication of the Society for Public Health Education, 46*(1), 146–156.

Logie, C., & Gibson, M. F. (2013). A mark that is no mark? Queer women and violence in HIV discourse. *Culture, Health & Sexuality, 15*(1), 29–43.

MacDonald, E. (1989). Theatre Rhinocerous: A gay company. *TDR, 33*(1), 79–93.

Martos, A. J. (2016). Vernacular knowledge and critical pedagogy: Conceptualising sexual health education for young men who have sex with men. *Sex Education, 16*(2), 184–198.

McClelland, S. I., & Fine, M. (2008). Writing on cellophane: Studying teen women's sexual desires, inventing methodological release points. In K. Gallagher (Ed.), *The methodological Dilemma: Creative, critical and collaborative approaches to qualitative research* (0th ed., pp. 259–288). London, UK: Routledge.

Michalak, E. E., Livingston, J. D., Maxwell, V., Hole, R., Hawke, L. D., & Parikh, S. V. (2014). Using theatre to address mental illness stigma: A knowledge translation study in bipolar disorder. *International Journal of Bipolar Disorders, 2*, 1.

UNAIDS. (2019). *Country: Eswatini*. UNAIDS, Geneva, Switzerland. Downloaded April 11, 2021 from: https://www.unaids.org/en/regionscountries/countries/swaziland

Wernick, L. J., Dessel, A. B., Kulick, A., & Graham, L. F. (2013). LGBTQQ youth creating change: Developing allies against bullying through performance and dialogue. *Children and Youth Services Review, 35*(9), 1576–1586.

Wernick, L. J., Woodford, M. R., & Kulick, A. (2014). LGBTQQ youth using participatory action research and theater to effect change: Moving adult decision-makers to create youth-centered change. *Journal of Community Practice, 22*(1–2), 47–66.

Chapter 6
Love, Intimate Inquiry and the Beloved Community

This chapter describes my experience working on a community-based study with internally displaced women in post-earthquake Haiti. The first section discusses the background to the project followed by lessons learned in the research process that signalled the salience of considering love for others as part of research. This is followed by a reflective conversation with CarolAnn Daniel, the study's co-principal investigator. A final section explores how researchers can integrate concepts of love, the beloved community, and intimate inquiry into their research practice.

6.1 Reflections on Learning with Internally Displaced Women in Post-Earthquake Haiti

One of the most compelling memories I have in learning about the power of community occurred during a study where we trained internally displaced women as peer health workers to deliver an HIV prevention program to other displaced women in Leogane, the epicentre of Haiti's 2010 earthquake. Peer health workers had named the project *Famn An Akyson Pou Sante Yo (FASY,* 'Women Taking Action for Their Health' in Kreyol). The premise was that peer health workers would deliver a six-week series of psychoeducational sessions to groups of 25 women. Peer health workers were diverse in age, ranging from their late teenage years to their early sixties, as well as in relationship status and education level. They all shared one thing in common: they had been displaced from their homes after the 2010 earthquake shook Leogane and destroyed 90% of its buildings.

I had never planned to work in Haiti. I was expecting to have a relaxing post-doctoral fellowship after completing my doctoral research in South India and dreamed of part-time work in coffee shops in Toronto while preparing manuscripts for publication. I had met CarolAnn Daniel several years before at a social work conference. She found me beside a poster I had prepared on HIV-related stigma and

C. Logie, *Working with Excluded Populations in HIV*, Social Aspects of HIV 8,
https://doi.org/10.1007/978-3-030-77048-8_6

shared her work with Caribbean migrants living with HIV in New York City who experienced the intersection of HIV-related stigma and racism. We kept in touch, collaborating the following year on a presentation in Jamaica at the Caribbean Studies Association. In October 2010, a few weeks after I defended my PhD thesis, I was at the same annual social work conference when CarolAnn found me again. Over lunch, she shared how she had been working in Haiti since the earthquake in January and thought that my HIV expertise could come in handy. A couple of months later, I saw a call for applications for early career investigators from Grand Challenges Canada. They were looking for "innovative" projects that would combine business, social and technological dimensions. I sent the call to CarolAnn, who immediately responded that I needed to fly to New York the next week as her colleagues from Leogane would be visiting and we could develop a grant proposal together.

I flew to New York, and spent a weekend sitting around a long kitchen table with a group of community workers who had started a youth development agency being operated out of metal shipping containers. We came up with the idea to hire women displaced from the earthquake and train them as peer health workers and combine this with an economic intervention to make peanut butter using solar power. This we hoped would reach the funder's requirements for social, business and technological innovation. To our great surprise we were funded.

From the start, there were many unanticipated challenges. Almost immediately someone stole the generator for electricity. The solar panels originally purchased for the project ended up playing a bigger role in powering the lights and the water pump for the agency and residents living in tents on the property. It was not financially feasible to include the planned for peanut butter component due to the high cost of electricity and insufficient solar energy.

We used tablets for the initial surveys we undertook to assess HIV knowledge, yet peer health workers and participants did not have smart phones and were not used to working with touch screens. The honorarium of five dollars, as small as we could make it to satisfy the research ethics protocol requirements, was more than the majority of participants made in one month. We had more than two hundred participants lining up to take part in the survey, some visibly emotional after receiving the five-dollar bill. We did not consider that the peer health workers might not feel confident, even after intensive training, to deliver a weekly intervention to twenty-five persons. So, together we decided to have peer health workers pair up to deliver the intervention, also helpful for intervention fidelity.

The intervention was conducted in the metal shipping containers, so participants ended up sitting on small furniture made for children. While we had originally imagined providing a snack and beverage halfway through the three-hour sessions, we soon learned that many women did not eat more than one meal per day, and if we provided the snack at the beginning of the session instead it helped participants focus. Another concern was the fact we excluded men. Each day when *FASY* meetings took place men would hang around the compound and ask when we would hold a program for them. These men described their challenges seeking employment, the stress of losing their homes, and wistfully remarked on how much fun the women seemed to be having.

The intervention involved training women displaced by the earthquake as peer health workers. Peer health workers helped to develop the *FASY* project curriculum, recruited other displaced women as participants, and facilitated group-based sessions. Topics addressed in these sessions included HIV and sexually transmitted infections, personal relationships, communication and decision making, mental health, resilience and coping, and creating community change. While initially conceptualized as a research project, FASY grew into much more than this, with peer health workers providing support to one another and to community members that lasted well beyond the scope of the project. For instance, peer health workers offered participants and other community members literacy classes, used their monthly wage to materially support their own family members (e.g., by building homes, paying school fees, purchasing equipment for practicing a trade). Peer health workers also provided emotional and social support to one another facilitating sessions, recruiting and retaining participants, and sharing advice and their own stories of navigating survival, mental health, and relationship challenges. Participants explained that by sharing stories of struggle and survival they experienced solidarity, gaining social support, happiness, and feelings of unity and togetherness.

Beyond the context of the intervention, the project helped me to reflect on the role of love and community. FASY peer health workers, from those aged eighteen to sixty, used their monthly stipend to take care of their families and to pay for their siblings or children's education. Visible bonds of togetherness included shared laughter between peer health workers and between peer health workers and participants throughout the intervention, including during times of illness and other hardship. A striking memory I have about the power of community occurred during a focus group. At the end of the project, we held focus groups to elicit feedback from participants. We mixed the focus groups to include participants from different peer health workers' groups, so that not all focus group participants knew one another. During one of the focus groups, a young woman, Roseline (a pseudonym) in her late teens broke down crying. Roseline explained that she was pregnant with her second child and her boyfriend had just left her. She felt hopeless, living in a tent with no work, and now needing to feed two children. An older woman sitting across the table, a stranger to her, looked and her and sharply stated (in Kreyol) "Sit up now! Dry your eyes!" I was shocked and looked at CarolAnn. She continued: "You are a strong woman. You don't need that boy. We have been there, in the place that you are. You can do this. We are here for you." The reaction was immediate. Evelyn stopped crying, dried her eyes and sat up taller. Other focus group members then described their own relationship difficulties and survival struggles, often as single parents navigating poverty. It was clear that Roseline was not alone, that people understood her suffering and recognized her strength. This example illustrates how love and solidarity can be integrated into struggles for personal and social transformation. The example also underscores the importance of creating space for persons with shared experiences and struggles to connect with one another in ways that foster relationships that increase individual and collective agency. Also notable to me in later reflective conversation with CarolAnn is the fact that she does not remember this moment from the focus group, although she was there alongside me co-facilitating. Memories and learning are personal and subjective, reinforcing the importance of recognizing multiple perspectives in order to better understand a phenomenon, and to reflect on the lessons learned from community-based research.

6.2 In Conversation: CarolAnn Daniel

*All names of persons except for CarolAnn Daniel and I have been changed for privacy.

Carmen: *I wanted to talk to you because I have been thinking of the power of FASY creating a platform for women to connect with each other. I wonder if it was the bonding between women in the groups. I think about the importance of creating spaces for people to connect like that. And that is when I started thinking about bell hooks and how she discusses the beloved community and how we actually take love out of research. I was wondering how you thought that love, solidarity or the beloved community might be relevant to how you experienced FASY.*

CarolAnn: *I feel like for me, I think it is always important to start to think about how spaces impact me. And what one of the biggest things I took away was, in fact, this meaning of community. For the very first time, I really felt that I was in a situation where although the personal relationships counted, that the community relationship was privileged above everything else. And I saw that at so many levels, both in the way people responded to me, but also in the way they responded to each other. There was just this sense of responsibility. And I guess perhaps at some point you can call it love that people had for each other that I had never seen before.*

And so, I just remember spending a lot of time thinking about all of the different conflicts that people were having, about all the little gossips. Always when something happened, people came together in such an amazing way. And that has always struck me, as that to me was transformational, both in terms of my own ideas about what it means to be in community as well as to see it in practice.

For example, I remember when Eveleyn's son caught some kind of stomach bug and he had to be hospitalized. I do not know if you remember that. And I just watched every day how people just came together to support her. They literally they had some woman who took her food. Then women were bringing clothes back to wash for her. Well, every day two people took turns, these moto's [motorcycle taxis] would come up to the yard every day. And all these guys would just jump on the moto with the food to take to the hospital because, you know, when we are in the hospital, you cannot leave people alone. They all came together to support her. Even as I was watching and I knew about all of these conflicts between her and the other girls in the yard. And I have never forgotten that. That was just amazing to me to see how every single person in the compound participated in helping her through this really difficult process when she thought her child was going to die. That was one thing that stayed with me.*

Another thing that actually stayed with me when I think about community in practice, there was once a young man that came to see Fabiola and the way he was dressed, I could see that he was a middle-class guy. I think he actually worked in one of the non-government agencies. And he came to the house to wait for Fabiola, and you know how she is in the morning. She takes her time getting dressed. And this young man is sitting in the outer vestibule waiting for her just very patiently, as people do in Haiti. And so, this this little naked boy comes running across the yard and he fell. And all of the dust and the dirt and all. And he is lying down and he is screaming. His face is all dirty and stuff, and he is not wearing any clothes, like the little kids are. And this guy dressed in a suit, got up, went out. And I am standing right there. He went past me, picked up the little boy. Took the handkerchief out of his pocket, wiped the kid's nose with his handkerchief and his face, then took his hands and dusted off his body. And then sent the kid on his way.*

I was just sitting there and just thinking. Right. What just happened here? I have never seen, first of all, a complete stranger respond to a little child like that. The fact is he was a man, coming from a place where masculinity is constructed not in this kind of caring way. So that was the other thing. And then this guy who was totally of a completely different social class, none of that mattered and he cared for this little boy. And I carry that image with me all the time of seeing this guy wiping the snotty nose of this little kid that he did not know.

Carmen: *I was thinking of this shared humanity that is central to the beloved community when you were talking. I thought about Fabiola* and how she let all of these people live in tents on her land. Our windows were mesh screens and I could hear, and I am sure you could too, people coughing in the tents outside my room. When you hear that it just felt very clear that we have this shared humanity.*

CarolAnn: *It is interesting that you that you mention that. We have had a lot of conflicts with Fabiola over the years, because I think that when we first arrived, she saw us as every other researcher. That researchers were coming with this idea that they know more about them than they know about themselves. For me, one of the ways that I was able to work through a lot of that was understanding her frustration, both with the system, with the lack of changes, and with all of the researchers circling in and out of Haiti, ourselves included. I was able to resolve that, because when I looked around and saw what she was doing, I thought that I understood it as a greater good than me. She had all these groups of people that she was basically feeding, her whole thing was to help each of these young people to find themselves meaningful work, to be able to be independent. And she was doing it solely on her own income, resources, and everything else. And she kept expanding and expanding it. It was the beloved community in practice, the way that people lived together, were forced to resolve conflicts, the way that the community was privileged beyond any of their personal relationships.*

Carmen: *For me, I have never experienced anything like that. I want to rewind because I also want to say it is funny having our memories together because it is more than just my memories. I do not know if you remember when we wrote the grant and how you said you have got to come to New York. All the folks from Leogane are going to be at (collaborator) house and we sat at the kitchen table for hours. We* *actually created the idea for FASY together and hammered out the design. I had never really experienced that level of engagement from so many people that were intimately connected with the community that we were working with from the beginning. I do not know why that is.*

CarolAnn: *We also became part of their lives and they became part of ours. I remember walking into town once with one of the young men who was banned from the compound because he had stolen something. And that to me also is just incredible. This idea that the worst punishment you can give to someone is to ban them. It speaks to the importance of community, that being apart from the community is like the worst thing that could happen to you. There were various people who were at some point asked to leave. And in everybody's eyes, that is the worst thing that can happen. I just remember walking into town once and coming back and we are running into this young man who had been kicked out of the compound for stealing something. And he walks me up to the gate. And the whole time we are walking he is saying, how is your family? How are the boys? And he remembered them by name. And so he walks me to the gate and he is still holding my hands. I realize at some point that I was going to have to say, "OK, I have to go now" because he is engaging me in conversation like he does not want to go. And I am aware that he is not able to come in. And it was just a really hard, difficult moment for me. I do not even remember if I was able to eat dinner that night. I remember going back to the house and thinking, oh, my God, I had to leave this guy outside. I wonder where he was going to eat dinner, where he was going to be. And here I am inside and there is all this food and I am eating and talking to everyone. And it did not feel okay.*

Now reflecting on it I think that is one of the ways that we at some point cease to be researchers and we were just part of this community. Of course, when that happens, I suppose you can bring in issues of objectivity and all of that. There are many ways that traditional research speaks to the separation. But I feel like some of the work that we did and the reason it was so successful, so impactful, is that we were able to break down those hierarchies and become part of this community.

Carmen: *I was not here for this, but I remember you saying that some of the women from the FASY groups were still meeting a year or so after our research ended.*

CarolAnn: *When I went back for my sabbatical, I guess it was a year later after we left, I interviewed some of the women who had participated [in FASY]. And two things that really, really struck me happened. One was that was one of the women that I interviewed said she admitted that she was still in the relationship that she realized was toxic and she was not able to leave it.*

She said to me, "Why? I could leave. But honestly, if I left, I am going back to a man who's going to be the same because they are all this way". And that was a very kind of sobering moment for me. In me saying, "how do you think that your relationships have evolved? Can you talk about that?" and she was like, "I am still in the same relationship. I am not proud of it, but they are all the same. If I left him, I would be going to a man who is pretty much the same."

So that left me thinking a lot. One of the questions I asked was "what do you think had the most impact on you from the FASY group?" And she said,

> *You know what? When I joined the group, I could not read. And I would go to community meetings and no one paid attention to me. No one. Nothing I said was valid. I always sat in the back. And I rarely ever raised my hands to say anything, because I knew I could not read. And everyone knew I could not read. And after I am learning to read. I became part of the reading group. But most importantly, when I go to the community forums now, I sit in the front. People now understand that I have knowledge about HIV. Everyone from the community, when we get on that topic, people come to me to talk about that. I feel so proud. That makes me feel like I am a respected part of the community now.*

I thought I have got to write about this. How sometimes when we go into a place, we think we are doing one thing. And in fact, sometimes what we are doing is not what communities need. People will take what it is that we are doing and find things that are meaningful for them. People take what they need, and you have to trust that and be okay with it. Because I went in with all these questions about the research and how did the research impact you. And she said the biggest takeaway for me is that now I am respected by the community. That was some of the findings that I had when I went back a year later.

Carmen: *What would you say to researchers who think that internally displaced people are hard to reach?*

CarolAnn: *For me, when I think about this, it really is not the people. It is the systems and the institutions for me that are the problem. And so, I think that the narrative that we have about people who need help is part of the problem. This idea that if you need help, that there is something wrong with you for your life being the way that it is. Like you are not able to get it together. Like you are not that intelligent, that you are not capable. Simply because in one aspect of your life, you may need help. And it is this very liberal idea of individualism that just creeps into everything that we do, that the ultimate goal is for all of us to be independent.*

Sometimes we need to think about our own stance and standpoints as it relates to these issues before we enter into spaces. I think that it is far easier to talk about people as a problem for them than it is to talk about systems and institutions. Because we ourselves need to feel like we are doing what is right, so long as we have someone to blame. It is not easy taking on an institution or a system. Quite frankly, we need a different set of skills in order to do that. And most of us do not have those skills. We do not understand how systems come together to create barriers for other people. Most of us are not familiar with that literature and cannot understand where to intervene. So, we basically blame the people that are the actual victims of these systems. I see this idea and this notion of "displaced" as being part of that "problematic" category.

Carmen: *Why do you think this idea of objectivity is so pervasive? We do not talk about love as a method or how love can be infused as part of interventions, not an intimate or romantic love, but a love that fuels social justice. What do you think about that? Because there is definitely some surprise, I think, when I bring it up in academic spaces.*

CarolAnn: *If I just think about from the social work perspective and a social science perspective, it is very much a white male, rational, liberal dominated sphere brain. This is where you come up with this idea that to be a good researcher is to be objective, to be removed from your 'subjects.' This suggests that you are separate from the 'subject', and the researcher is usually seen as much more capable, intelligent and so forth. Clearly, I think people always feel it—and certainly communities of colour feel it—when people come in with this idea that I know more about you than you know about yourself. This concept of objectivity is infused in social science. That is what we have all learned, so that is how we understand both ourselves and the world, but also that is how we are rewarded. If you do research that does not prove that you have been objective then people do not think your work is legitimate. So, for many of us who want to move away from that, it is difficult if you also want to be successful. In many ways, we are asked to make choices: a career as a respected researcher or as a career as a researcher who is really engaging with people from this perspective of oneness, wholeness or togetherness.*

I am also thinking about in my book project this concept of radical love. That is the love of others, even as they are hating you. How do you actively be engaged with people who have no regard for you? I am thinking that there is just no way to get around this work unless we begin to think about both a radical kind of self-love, but also radical love of community. Some of the work that I am doing on myself is like, how do I engage with these people who are haters in a loving way, even as I am protecting myself from someone spewing on me? That was a little aside, but I think it is the idea. We are not rewarded for thinking about this, for moving beyond the boundaries of our disciplines.

Carmen: *This idea of loving people even when they seem to hate you seems so powerful. I was doing a focus group a couple of weeks ago with some transgender women in Jamaica who were experiencing homelessness and living with HIV. They really started acting in challenging ways, playing music and videos on their phone in the middle of the focus group, taking phone calls, having side conversations, and would not listen to myself or the other facilitators in trying to be respectful and focused. They were arguing with one another. It was a chaotic mess. At the break I went upstairs to clear my head. I then realized they were 'acting out' like teenagers, trying to push myself and the others from the community agency away from them. Almost like they wanted us to dislike them and push them away, because that is what they were used to.*

CarolAnn: *If I may just turn the lens, the camera, back on us a little bit. Is it possible that they feel like there is nothing that they really have to say that is respected or is going to be taken seriously because they had situations like that in the past? And so, for them, this coming together was not any different from experiences of where people said they would do this or other research. That nothing happened to benefit them.*

Carmen: *I agree. I think you are right. I was asking them what adherence barriers they had because that was the grant focus. That was not their priority. People were saying they did not have enough food to take with their meds. They have to work all night largely doing sex work. They felt sick after taking the meds so could* *not take them before going to work, but also did not want to take them when they came back to sleep because it gave them nightmares. They want food and they want accommodation. HIV is actually not their priority right now. I was off of their priorities. They all talked about food but as a researcher, that is not something I could provide other than one meal during the focus group. I struggled with that.*

CarolAnn: *That is the point. And that is the policy. I cannot give life. You see what it is like. The thing that they want most, you are not able to give to them. And they are aware of that. So, they are asking, "Why am I here? Just give me the money. I have heard this before. You know, none of this is making any difference to me." This is why I want to bring it back to the Haiti situation. It is another reason why I find it difficult thinking about working in Haiti today because so much of what they need I feel like we cannot provide.*

Carmen: *It is beyond research, it is actual structural and economic interventions with employment and housing and food that is needed. In low-income countries like Haiti the government maybe cannot afford to take care of everybody.*

CarolAnn: *The fact of the matter is beyond that. Even the structures in Haiti, the government as it is currently conceptualized, does not work for them. It does not keep them safe. It does not help to feed them. It does not help to provide health care and all of the things that people need to stay intact. And I think this is why community is so important for this group of people that we worked with.*

Carmen: *I remember that idea of reciprocity came up in our focus groups with youth. We asked the youth about their dreams for the future. A lot of them said "I want to give back and help others." Remember when the FASY peer health workers used their salary to build a house for their family or pay for their siblings to go to school. There was a feeling like this money is not just for me, but to help my community.*

CarolAnn: *Absolutely. The biggest thing I got from that is how much the community is privileged above all other types of relationships, including romantic relationships. We saw it in so many different ways. People were really concerned about what others thought about their community. People wanted to be part of the community. Everything was about was 'we' and 'us.' And even when they talked about wanting things for themselves, it was to further help the community.*

Carmen: *I wanted to ask you, what lessons do you think that this reflection on our work and on love, community solidarity, can inform the next researcher or the person who is going to read about this? How can they use this to move forward?*

CarolAnn: *You talked about this when we were planning the grant. And I think it is what we have to work on. First of all, this idea of working on people individually is something that we have to find ways to put aside. One of the things that we need to begin to privilege in our work is the importance of the interdependence of ideas and people. So that the question is not what do you need as an individual to take care of yourself, but what does your community need in order to take care of you and its members? There is a kind of interdependency, as well as more of an uplifting of the community. I think sometimes as researchers, we go in with this individual lens and we are looking at individual people. Perhaps we need to start thinking about people in community and the interdependence that is necessary in order for that to work.*

Centering our work around that, because I think it would force you to ask different questions, to think about life and the issues differently. I think that is definitely one lesson that I learned from Haiti. And one that I think would be helpful to me in any research I did going forward.

Carmen: *I have to tell this story because I learned so much from this. I do this talk in arts-based research methods as an example of how important it is to listen to community and I share my own mistakes as an example. I remember we made a video for FASY on HIV information, and they put together this video and they added footage from the children playing soccer outside, the bus ride, the chickens and roosters, and people cooking. I watched it said: "this is way too long, you guys need to cut all of the background stuff." But we decided to show it to the FASY peer workers before making changes and they loved it. They said the best part was the background, and that is what is going to make people want to watch the part of the video with the HIV information. This is their community, and they literally wanted to see the context that they were living in represented before going to the research focus on HIV. It was such a lesson for me.*

CarolAnn: *They were enraptured with seeing themselves in the conversation. That is another important piece for researchers—help your participants to see themselves in the narrative of what you do. Coming back to this idea of a loving community. We told FASY participants they could bring their immediate family members to the ceremony to celebrate the end of FASY and entire villages came. Over a thousand people came. I think even people who did not have anyone in the program, the entire village came. That is not a lie. If this example is not about realizing the importance of community, I do not know what is. It was just incredible. What I loved about the work in Haiti and what was going on when I think about it, is how they kept helping us understand what to do. They were coming to us and saying, wow, I think people would respond if you did this. They were always trying to help us to be more successful. They saw the importance of the work and wanted their community to be helped by it.*

6.3 Love, Intimate Inquiry and the Beloved Community

> A love ethic presupposes that everyone has the right to be free, to live fully and well. To bring a love ethic to every dimension of our lives, our society would need to embrace change…We do this by choosing to work with individuals we admire and respect; by committing to give our all to relationships; by embracing a global vision wherein we see our lives and our fate as intimately connected to those of everyone else on the planet (p. 87, hooks, 2001).

This quotation synthesizes several themes and examples discussed in the reflective conversation with CarolAnn. For instance, the focus on collective belonging and wellbeing as central to community wellbeing, beyond a focus on the individual, underscores an understanding of our interconnectedness and the ways in which our wellbeing may be realized through our relations with others. This section will explore how love can inform a research approach with persons who may be categorized as hard to reach.

6.3.1 *Conceptualizing Love*

Love has been conceptualized in many ways (Sternberg, 2013). Early psychological models developed by Robert Sternberg and Susan Grajek in the USA focused on the convergence of social bonds, emotions, motivation, and cognitions (Sternberg & Grajek, 1984). These bonds include trust, respect and caring, among others. Shortly thereafter Sternberg posited a triangular theory of love that included intimacy (feelings of being close and connected), passion (drive, attraction and excitement) and commitment (choosing to begin and maintain love) (Sternberg, 1986). He then conceptualized a third approach to love; in this approach, love is understood and being created through narrative, and thus love is in fact a story (Sternberg, 1995). The myriad ways in which stories are shared through lived experience, between friends and family, and the media produce expectations and ideas about love (Sternberg, 1995). Bringing these together, it is clear that our understandings of love are produced in the interplay between personal characteristics, the socio-cultural environment, and common interests. Flexibility, wisdom, intelligence and creativity help us to adapt to and navigate changes in relationships over time (Sternberg, 2013). That said, most of these approaches to love focus on persons in intimate relationships, with less focus on love in the context of research.

By pausing for a moment to think, as researchers we can become more aware of our own stories about relationships and love—and how we apply these stories to our relationships with colleagues and participants, and in our everyday lives. To do this we may reflect on the ways that our personalities and our histories shaped the way we view love and, in turn, how we experience relationships of caring and trust. For instance, in reflective conversation with CarolAnn, I considered my understanding that emerged from conducting a focus group with disinterested participants. My initial understanding of the interaction was based on my experience as a social worker learning about some clients' rejection sensitivity; some people may expect to be rejected and as a result engage in practices to push others away. My interpretation of the events created a story in which I situated the issue the focus group participants were experiencing as one of social exclusion, but also one that stressed the importance of connecting with myself as a researcher. However, CarolAnn's reflection on my interpretation signalled the need for me to consider social justice more deeply within the context in which the experience occurred. My research focus on adherence to antiretroviral therapy did not align with participants' priorities and needs. The participants knew I could not meet their priorities and therefore disengaged. The importance of the researcher-participant connection therefore does not outweigh the importance of research that aligns with community needs. People can be experienced as 'hard to reach' when the research focus overlooks their personal and collective priorities.

Other definitions of love stress a focus on our shared humanity. For instance, Ancient Greek philosophy distinguishes between eros (romantic love), filia (brotherly and interpersonal love), and agape (love for one's community) (Brosi & hooks, 2012). Yet these forms of love are often conceptualized as separate, with romantic/erotic love privileged in Western, more individualistic societies. And separating our interpersonal/intimate and community lives can overlook the role that interdependence plays in producing empathy both for ourselves and for others. A conceptualization of love as "the material and conceptual pursuit of our own or someone else's humanity" (Laura, 2016, p. 215) is particularly salient for understanding how HIV researchers can work from a place of love. There is also a history, notably in the tradition of Paulo Freire, of viewing love as central to our humanity and a key ingredient in our work to deconstruct and dismantle social hierarchy (Darder, 2017).

bell hooks (2001), among others, has discussed the importance of the values that a *love ethic* imparts, including yet extending beyond intimate relationships. These values include openness and honesty, integrity, loyalty and commitment. In line with such an ethic, the nurturing of wellbeing takes precedence over career and material gain. Informed by such a love ethic, the ways that people can challenge different forms of marginalization include embracing new perspectives and taking action to advance social justice. Tellingly, hooks reminds us that "all the great movements for social justice in our society have strongly emphasized a love ethic" (hooks, 2001, p. xix). Such an approach requires radical change and dismantling oppressive and exclusionary systems such as patriarchy. Research informed by a love ethic can enrich the lives of ourselves and others through the co-production of knowledge to reshape thoughts, words and actions.

Yet fear of love is often embedded within socio-cultural norms and can undergird resistance to change. This also holds true in research. Love as a research method and love as data may seem at odds with the dominant positivist expectations that researchers should be detached and objective (Laura, 2010, 2013). Grounding research in love and relationships, as CarolAnn described, can feel like making a choice between research success and obscurity. In social and academic contexts where love is feared and devalued, hooks reminds us of the courage required to change our perspective to explore the relevance of love to our research and practice. Not only can change invoke fear, but challenging our stories and underlying narratives about love and the relevance to our research practice can be personally and academically difficult as it questions the binary division between attached/detached and personal/academic.

6.3.2 Conceptualizing the Beloved Community

> Agape is disinterested love. It is a love in which the individual seeks not his own good, but the good of his neighbor. Agape does not begin by discriminating between worthy and unworthy people, or any qualities people possess. It begins by loving others for their sakes. It

is an entirely "neighbor-regarding concern for others," which discovers the neighbor in every man it meets. Therefore, agape makes no distinction between friends and enemy; it is directed toward both (King, 1986).

The roots of the term *beloved community* can be traced back to the USA-based philosopher Josiah Royce (1855–1916) and to the African American Baptist minister, activist and Civil Rights Movement leader Martin Luther King Jr. (1929–1968), among others (Herstein, 2009). Royce conceptualized the beloved community as persons with a dedicated commitment to shared values and principles. To realize such a community, Royce underscored the need to practice kindness, patience and courage, among other virtues. King (1958) later took up the term beloved community as part of the Six Principles of Non-Violence, in which he envisioned that non-violent conflict resolution between persons and society would contribute to the development a beloved community centered on principles of love.

As defined in the opening quotation of this section, the type of love that King believed was critical to developing a beloved community was *agape*. King explained that "agape is not a weak, passive love. It is love in action. Agape is love seeking to preserve and create community" (King, 1991, p. 20). Attaining the beloved community in this perspective requires persistent effort and struggle. Extending Royce's conceptualization of the beloved community, King added justice, non-violence, anti-racism, and love as central to the pursuit of community. He believed that justice initiatives, such as intergroup dialogue and collaboration, could reduce violence and transform oppressive and hierarchical systems. Also central to King's work was embracing the contributions of African American culture with pride while challenging racism (King, 2012, The King Center, 2020).

Other writers and activists, including bell hooks (2000) and Grace Lee Boggs, later wrote about the concept of the beloved community and its liberatory potential. Shared principles in their writing include a focus on relationships between people working for change; community as the change agent; the importance of belonging; radical openness; and accountability. Also central to the concept of the beloved community is the idea that conflict is natural, and that love and justice can overcome conflict through the use of strategies such as dialogue and nonviolence. hooks called for special attention to the practical means by which the beloved community could produce changes in thought and action (hooks, 2003). Grace Lee Boggs and Scott Kurashige (2012) similarly gave a focus to action: "we urgently need to bring to our communities the limitless capacity to love, serve, and create for and with each other" (p. 47).

The concept of beloved community in practice was informed by Boggs' activism in *humanity stretching movements*, including her work within the movements for civil rights, labour rights, women's rights, Asian American rights, Black Power, and environmental justice. This activism led to an understanding of the need to rethink and rebuild human relationships to foster self and structural transformations to transform anger into productive change. In particular, Boggs and Kurashige (2012) aimed to reframe perspectives toward the city of Detroit. Perceived by outsiders as dangerous, decaying, and destructive, Detroit could also be viewed as holding the possibility for radical change through grassroots local activism. For instance, urban farming could spark values such as cooperation and respect. Building critical connections can create and sustain movements. Community building also deepens understanding of the "web of interconnected social movements" (Juan, 2015, p. 92). A concern for shared humanity may be leveraged to build coalitions between identity-based social movements to advance social change. Boggs frequently asked the question "what time is it on the clock of the world" (Boggs & Kurashige, 2012, p. 18) to generate dialogue about the connections between people (persons across the globe) and time (between our actions now and their future impacts). Knowing a *place* reflects a consciousness that engenders understanding of historical and current local priorities and issues.

Boggs and others saw the beloved community as inclusive of the horizontal relationships between people working for change. Conflict resolution from a beloved community perspective is grounded in non-violence and the recognition that identifying and implementing approaches to solving conflict can deepen relationships (Juan, 2015). Brosi and hooks (2012) also discussed how conflict is central to community building, and how a commitment to the beloved community can help people develop conflict resolution strategies. Our understanding of conflict is also influenced by perceptions of the 'other,' and how much we believe those we are in conflict with are worthy of dignity, respect, and redemption. Situating ourselves within a beloved community of practice (including HIV research) requires us to grapple with our relationships and conflicts with others while working for social justice.

An expansive view of the beloved community includes both the goals and processes of research:

> The beloved community defines the relationships among those working for change and also the desired results of these efforts. In other words, those of us working for institutional change endeavor to become a beloved community among ourselves as we are striving for all of society to exemplify the beloved community (Brosi & hooks, 2012, p. 76).

In the beloved community, everyone has the capacity to change and transform. From this perspective, conversations with others with differing viewpoints can be grounded in a new way of communication that is inclusive rather than rooted in domination (Brosi & hooks, 2012). Communication can therefore be a tool for meaningfully engaging with multiple perspectives. For instance, CarolAnn described the power of community in holding collective responsibility to provide care and support for one another. She also explained that when people broke the community's trust, such as by stealing, they lost what was most important to them—their place in community. In contexts such as in post-earthquake Haiti, community rejection had particularly harsh consequences. The local community was powerful: it offered connection and survival support yet could also be punishing and unforgiving for those who transgressed norms. The concept of the beloved community includes engagement, struggle, and openness. Being in community with others necessitates learning about one another. And knowing one another includes learning about painful, disappointing, or otherwise uncomfortable things (Brosi & hooks, 2012).

For instance, socio-economic, gender, racial and other power differences can create tension and conflict. Negotiating fear of the 'other' and discomfort with perceived difference is thus a key element of building community, as is the ability to pursue reconciliation. When we are unwilling or unable to negotiate these differences and interrogate privilege, the "dominator culture" hooks described (2003, p. 197) will persist.

A beloved community perspective on epidemics should include the multiple perspectives—both public health and faith based—that advance a common vision of wellbeing for the most vulnerable. However, the dominance of academic perspectives often shuts out community and other non-academic perspectives including those of faith-based groups, overlooking their success in community mobilization and engagement. Part of this success in mobilizing communities derives from the use of narrative approaches, such as storytelling, to manage health crises including HIV in faith communities (Ransome et al., 2018). To enact beloved community principles in health research and practice, researchers need to meaningfully engage with community expertise and connectedness. At the same time, community leaders should leverage an ethics of care with a focus on the most vulnerable. Warren et al. (2011) describe that "while the notion of the Beloved Community may seem idealistic, so does the vision of public health" (p. 12). The beloved community is germane to HIV research that has a long history rooted in activism and community engagement. The *Denver Principles* developed in 1983 in the USA by a group of people living with HIV created a statement from the Advisory Committee of People with AIDS that called for dignity and respect (Advisory Committee of the People with AIDS, 1983). These Principles included the following "Recommendations for all people":

1. Support and membership in our struggle against those who would fire us from our jobs, evict us from our homes, refuse to touch us or separate us from our loved ones, our community or our peers, since available evidence does not support the view that AIDS can be spread by casual, social contact.
2. Not scapegoat people with AIDS, blame us for the epidemic or generalize about our lifestyles.

The Canadian HIV activist Jessica Lynn Whitbread has applied concepts of community building in her HIV research and activism. For instance, her project 'Tea Time: Mapping Informal Networks of Women Living with HIV' involved hosting tea parties with women living with HIV in Canada and documenting participation with personalized letters and teacups[1]. *Love Positive Women* is an annual community building initiative started by Jessica in 2012 that takes place every February 1–14. She describes *Love Positive Women's (LPW)* focus on love and community:

> Using Valentine's Day as a backdrop, LPW creates a platform for individuals and communities to engage in public and private acts of love and caring for women living with HIV.

---

[1]To learn more about Jessica Whitbread's master thesis "Tea Time: Mapping Informal Networks of Women Living with HIV" see: http://jessicawhitbread.com/project/tea-time/.

> Going beyond romantic love to deep community love and social justice, LPW is call to action. It requires participants to reflect on how they as either a woman living with HIV or an ally will commit to loving women living with HIV and then do it. Through action, change can be made to fueling economies of love and compassion. Working from a place of strength, LPW focuses on the idea of interconnectedness, relationship building, loving oneself and loving one's community. (From Jessica Lynn Whitbread's website's project statement on Love Positive Women[2]).

How might HIV research look different if it was informed by principles from the beloved community and the Denver Principles? For instance, Auerbach and Hoppe (2015) discuss the need for HIV researchers to expand perspectives on pre-exposure prophylaxis (PrEP) beyond "getting drugs into bodies" to understand the complex and changing social dynamics surrounding PrEP. Framing PrEP within beloved community principles could allow an exploration of the synergy between individual, relational, and community perspectives that could construct PrEP as a tool to balance self-protection and community wellbeing. Regaining a shared ethics of love and care in HIV research requires more than a focus on relationships. Values matter, as does putting aside differences for a common goal and investing time into acts of care.

6.3.3 Intimate Inquiry

Laura (2010, 2013) conceptualizes *intimate inquiry* as a research method wherein we are explicit about our own positionality as researchers with connections to the topic and/or participants. An intimate inquiry approach recognizes that research has real-life consequences for people's lives—including the researcher's own life. The researcher's passion and motivation driving their work is connected to personal, social and relational contexts—and these connections should be made transparent (Laura, 2013). An intimate inquiry approach is grounded in *love acts* that view all persons as interconnected and deserving of freedom. Laura (2010) describes how research grounded in loving practice can guide the way we 'do' research, as manifested in our thoughts, words and actions, and shape the knowledge that is produced. This way of doing research is not focused on the 'unknown' participant, but rather is approached as a caring, kind, and thoughtful practice such as how we would treat our loved ones. Love conceptualized as non-romantic actions that are humanizing and empowering (Laura, 2013) can inform research approaches with persons categorized as hard to reach.

This person-centered approach in intimate inquiry acknowledges researchers' personal perspectives toward issues and people that drive their work to improve wellbeing. Paradoxically, researchers often actively conceal any intimate connection between themselves and their research (Daza, 2008). As Laura (2010) explained: "Love, many would argue, has got nothing to do with this [research]" (p. 281). This

[2]The Love Positive Women statement available here: http://jessicawhitbread.com/project/love-positive-women/.

tension between intimate inquiry and traditional, 'objective' research mirrors the history of undervaluing qualitative research in comparison to quantitative research (Denzin, 2007). It also reflects CarolAnn's discussion about the way in which qualitative research that integrates love and care can be seen as less rigorous and scientific. Yet this qualitative-quantitative divide is undergoing change (Braun & Clarke, 2019), in part due to an understanding of the heterogeneity of methods within each approach (Allwood, 2012). Researchers guided by a love ethic navigate a precarious balance between intimate inquiry and academic legitimacy when developing research questions and methods. Embracing intimate inquiry requires consideration of a wide range of issues, including negotiating ethical dilemmas; identifying research foci, including personal, social, intellectual and methodological dimensions; exploring personal and social worlds; situating the researcher and their values, purpose, and assumptions; and self-reflection (Laura, 2010). Three main methods in intimate inquiry include: witnessing, engaging, and working in solidarity with and for communities.

Exploring love in social research signals the importance of care. Laura (2013) describes *witnessing* as an approach that demonstrates love in research. This is an approach that involves thoughtfully listening, seeing, and noticing people in a deliberate way in order to understand and validate their stories and what they believe is meaningful. In this way "the act of witnessing is an invitation to pay attention, to reflect, to learn about lived lives" (Laura, 2013, p. 290). The act of witnessing is particularly salient to amplify visibility among persons who experience marginalization and public indifference. Witnessing can also be applied to the example discussed earlier in the chapter, where the young pregnant woman in the focus group was supported by the other focus group members when she broke down crying. The other women validated her story and struggle, as well as her strength. Witnessing a person's lived experiences—both joyful and painful—can affirm humanity. Love-based approaches to research are predicated on empathy and responsibility to advance social justice.

Engaging refers to identifying the challenges and complexities in the social world. This requires dialogue and deliberation to explore topics that seem commonplace and others that are taboo. This dialogue involves discussion regarding what was witnessed from multiple standpoints. The aim of individual and collective engagement is liberation through increased understanding of, and capacity to address, inequities and social change. From a love-focused perspective, courageous engagement requires constructing narratives to share the research process and findings in ways that reflect empathy and spark new understandings of the social world (Laura, 2016). As CarolAnn and I discussed in reflective conversation, it was important for peer health workers and participants to recognize themselves, their stories and their environment in a video about the research project which we made.[3] CarolAnn described how when viewing it, participants: "were enraptured with

[3]Famn an Aksyon Pou Sante Yo (FASY) video https://www.youtube.com/watch?v=YxjJ5dAtEmA.

seeing themselves in the conversation. That is another important piece for researchers—help your participants to see themselves in the narrative of what you do."

Finally, intimate inquiry is grounded in *solidarity*, whereby researchers collaborate meaningfully with participants in a research journey (Laura, 2010). Research following principles of solidarity focuses on shared objectives and priorities between the researchers and the researched, to ensure research processes and outcomes align with community values, principles, and hospitality (Denzin, 2007). From a perspective of solidarity, research is a service conducted with and for others. The researcher practising intimate inquiry understands the potential consequences of their research—both positive and negative—for real persons with hopes, lives, dreams and relationships (Laura, 2010). This approach guides researchers to consider collective—rather than only individual—approaches to research questions. Research participants should be understood as co-constructors of knowledge, particularly when engaged in determining the focus of the research. An approach rooted in solidarity invites researchers to build connections within the communities they are working with and leverage resources to meet community needs (Denzin, 2007; Martin & Glesne, 2002).

The concept of hospitality is a cornerstone of solidarity. In community-based projects, researchers are often welcomed into various spaces including homes, places of worship, and community centers, among others, and often with food, music and celebration. Social practices of hospitality extend beyond this however—they include providing others with the sense of belonging to community (Martin & Glesne, 2002). Practising from an ethic of hospitality can guide researchers to share more of ourselves, to provide food and comfort in the research process, as well as share the knowledge that is co-produced (Denzin, 2007). This concept of hospitality and sharing was clear in CarolAnn's description of the research knowledge mobilization event, when study participants brought family and village members together to hear the results from the study and watch the video:

> Coming back to this idea of a loving community. We told FASY participants they could bring their immediate family members to the ceremony to celebrate the end of FASY and entire villages came. Over a thousand people came. I think even people who did not have anyone in the program, the entire village came... If this example is not about realizing the importance of community, I do not know what is.

Hospitality is a community-level practice that may be offered by individuals but resides within larger social networks and social worlds. Researchers too can endeavour to offer hospitality to communities we engage with.

Taken together, an intimate inquiry approach offers researchers the opportunity to be more transparent about their work, what their connection is to community, and to develop and grow this connection in line with the priorities of communities they are working for. Doing so, raises the question whether if we were to apply an approach of witnessing, engaging, and solidarity, would we be more likely to find persons labelled hard to reach? Ultimately, the practice of research can also be understood as a practice of love, similar to Freire's conceptualization of teaching: "I understand the process of teaching as an act of love…it is an act of love as an expression of good care, a need to love first of what you do…in loving the very teaching process I cannot exclude loving those I work with when teaching, and those whom I teach" (Freire; cited in Leistyna, 2004, p. 27). Research guided by a love ethic invites us to approach colleagues and participants with the care and respect we would give to our kin, and mobilize research findings for improving their wellbeing.

6.4 Rethinking Hard to Reach Through Love, Beloved Community and Intimate Inquiry

This chapter has explored the power of community that was key to survival and belonging among people we worked with displaced by Haiti's 2010 earthquake. The case example working with internally displaced women underscores, as in each of the previous chapters, the importance of developing research with and for communities to address their priorities and harness their strengths. An intimate inquiry approach to research can facilitate building and sustaining community connection by encouraging us to be transparent about why we are doing research and identifying our connection with the topic and communities. Witnessing, engaging, and working in solidarity are but some of the ways in which we can practice love in our research. The concept of forgiveness is also central to the concept of a beloved community in which there is space and belief that all persons can change and transform. Researchers may consider this concept of forgiveness in our personal and professional lives when persons seemingly disappoint us and let us down—including research participants, persons we experience as hard to reach, and ourselves and colleagues when we make mistakes. We can also expand our vision of love beyond one of intimacy to one of a shared humanity to guide our commitment to work with and for communities to advance social justice. An ethic of love premised on our interconnectedness can help us to rethink and dismantle the hierarchies that might otherwise exist between researchers and participants.

Key to the beloved community is conceptualizing alternative ways of knowing, being, and relating through practising *radical openness*. hooks described this as follows: "this space of radical openness is a margin—a profound edge. Locating oneself there is difficult yet necessary. It is not a 'safe place'" (hooks, 1989, p. 19). Being radically open requires seeing both the centre and the margin, and understanding the margin as a site of resistance. In practice, radical openness is nonjudgmental and non-blaming, listens to voices of persons different from ourselves, and respects difference (Brosi & hooks, 2012). It also requires the ability to change one's mind upon the receipt of new information and ideas (hooks, 2003). As a research method, radical openness requires courage and humility to seek out multiple perspectives to enhance understanding of a phenomenon. It includes an understanding that multiple perspectives are necessary because all methods (and researchers) have flaws and blind spots. Rather than striving for definitive truth or answers, researchers apply their own interpretations to the data. Research guided by radical openness is better positioned to accept and learn from uncertainty and ambiguity without feeling the need to hold on to established theories (Wolch, 2003).

The concept of the beloved community can inform the way we see not only participants but research teams, and the ways we manage conflict in our lives to consider balancing love and justice to build healthy communities. CarolAnn described how "this idea that the worst punishment you can give to someone is to ban them. It speaks to the importance of community." Although a core tenet of the beloved community is forgiveness, she recalls the situation whereby a young man was banished from the compound we were working and living on for stealing. Young people were banished from the compound for stealing on several occasions during our study. This example demonstrates how lack of forgiveness occurred simultaneously with deep caring. Community members watched out for one another and took care of one another in difficult times, reflecting the concern for neighbours that is central to the concept of a beloved community. The values and principles underpinning a beloved community may therefore be complex—sometimes caring and sometimes unforgiving—as communities may be forced to make difficult decisions to balance self-protection with community wellbeing.

Taken together the approaches discussed in this chapter aim to build healthy, loving, and just communities. Applying an intimate inquiry approach that carefully embraces love in our research methods foregrounds the impact of research on real people. This does not erase the complexity in our studies, disallow presenting negative findings, ignore conflict, or allow guilt for power imbalances between researchers and participants to impede the formation of authentic connections (Domínguez, 2000). Instead, it offers us new perspectives with which to explore community-level issues and collective experiences, and encourages us to situate ourselves within communities that nurture and foster growth, insight and social change. This approach holds promise for engaging socially excluded communities who could be categorized as hard to reach. As hooks (2003) describes below, love is one of the key means by which we can reduce the gap with the 'other':

> When I come here, or to any place and feel myself to be somehow not fully present or seen, what allows me to enter this space of otherness is love. It is the love that I can generate within myself, as a light and send out, beam out, that can touch people. Love can bridge the sense of otherness. It takes practice to be vigilant, to beam that love out. It takes work (p. 162).

References

Advisory Committee of the People with AIDS. (1983). *The denver principles.* Downloaded February 28, 2021 from: https://actupny.org/documents/Denver.html

Allwood, C. M. (2012). The distinction between qualitative and quantitative research methods is problematic. *Quality & Quantity, 46*(5), 1417–1429.

Auerbach, J. D., & Hoppe, T. A. (2015). Beyond "getting drugs into bodies": Social science perspectives on pre-exposure prophylaxis for HIV. *Journal of the International AIDS Society, 18*(4S3), 19983.

Boggs, G. L., & Kurashige, S. (2012). *The next American revolution: Sustainable activism for the twenty-first century*. Berkeley, California, USA: University of California Press.

Braun, V., & Clarke, V. (2019). Novel insights into patients' life-worlds: The value of qualitative research. *The Lancet Psychiatry, 6*(9), 720–721.

Brosi, G., & hooks, b. (2012). The beloved community: A conversation between bell hooks and George Brosi. *Appalachian Heritage, 40*(4), 76–86.

Darder, A. (2017). *Reinventing Paulo Freire: A pedagogy of love* (2nd ed.). New York, USA: Routledge.

Daza, S. L. (2008). Decolonizing researcher authenticity. *Race Ethnicity and Education, 11*(1), 71–85.

Denzin, N. K. (Ed.). (2007). *Ethical futures in qualitative research: Decolonizing the politics of knowledge*. Walnut Creek, CA: Left Coast Press.

Domínguez, V. R. (2000). For a politics of love and rescue. *Cultural Anthropology, 15*(3), 361–393.

Herstein, G. (2009). The Roycean roots of the beloved community. *The Pluralist, 4*(2), 91–107.

hooks, b. (1989). Choosing the margin as a space of radical openness. *Framework: The Journal of Cinema and Media, 36*, 15–23.

hooks, b. (2001). *All about love: New visions (first perennial edition)*. New York: Harper Perennial.

hooks, b. (2003). *Teaching community: A pedagogy of hope*. Boca Raton, Florida: Routledge.

Juan, K. A.-S. (2015). "We are extraordinarily lucky to be living in these times": A conversation with grace lee Boggs. *Frontiers: A Journal of Women Studies, 36*(2), 92–123.

King, M. L, Jr. 1929–1968. (1958). *Stride toward freedom; the Montgomery story*. New York: Harper & Row.

King, M. L. (1986). An experiment in love. In *A testament of hope: The essential writings of Martin Luther King, Jr* (1st ed., pp. 16–20). New York, USA: HarperOne.

King, M. L. (1991). *A testament of hope: The essential writings and speeches of Martin Luther King, Jr* (J. M. Washington, ed.; 1st Harper Collins pbk. ed). HarperOne, New York, USA.

King, M. L. (2012). *A gift of love: Sermons from strength to love and other preachings*. London, UK: Penguin Books.

Laura, C. T. (2010). Home/work: Engaging the methodological dilemmas and possibilities of intimate inquiry. *Race Ethnicity and Education, 13*(3), 277–293.

Laura, C. T. (2013). Intimate inquiry: Love as "data" in qualitative research. *Cultural Studies ↔ Critical Methodologies, 13*(4), 289–292.

Laura, C. T. (2016). Intimate inquiry: A love-based approach to qualitative research. *Critical Questions in Education, 7*(3), 215–231.

Leistyna, P. (2004). Presence of mind in the process of learning and knowing: A dialogue with Paulo Freire. *Teacher Education Quarterly, 31*(1), 17–29.

Martin, P. M., & Glesne, C. (2002). From the Global Village to the Pluriverse? 'Other' ethics for cross-cultural qualitative research. *Ethics, Place & Environment, 5*(3), 205–221.

Ransome, Y., Bogart, L. M., Nunn, A. S., Mayer, K. H., Sadler, K. R., & Ojikutu, B. O. (2018). Faith leaders' messaging is essential to enhance HIV prevention among black Americans: Results from the 2016 National Survey on HIV in the black community (NSHBC). *BMC Public Health, 18*(1), 1392.

Sternberg, R. (1986). A triangular theory of love. *Psychological Review, 93*(2), 119–135.

Sternberg, R. (1995). Love as a story. *Journal of Social and Personal Relationships, 12*(4), 541–546.

Sternberg, R. (2013). Searching for love. *The Psychologist, 26*(2), 98–101.

Sternberg, R., & Grajek, S. (1984). The nature of love. *Journal of Personality and Social Psychology, 47*(2), 312–329.

The King Center. (2020). The King philosophy. *The King Center*. https://thekingcenter.org/king-philosophy/

Warren, R. C., Walker, B., Maclin, S. D., Miles-Richardson, S., Tarver, W., & James, C. M. (2011). Respecting and protecting the beloved community, especially susceptible and vulnerable populations. *Journal of Health Care for the Poor and Underserved, 22*(3 Suppl), 3–13.

Wolch, J. R. (2003). Radical openness as method in urban geography. *Urban Geography, 24*(8), 645–646.

Chapter 7
Conclusions and Moving Forward

Throughout this book the aim has been to expand the reader's methodological imagination so as to inspire both "courage and intellectual stretch" (p. 459, Fine, 2007) regarding how we see—or overlook—persons labelled hard to reach. The focus has been on exploring possibilities for transforming research practice to better engage with excluded populations. The goal has been to disrupt the dominant narrative that some persons are hard to reach, and instead offer new perspectives and approaches to such work grounded in hope, solidarity, community strengths, creativity and context. Each chapter has taken a community-based research study conducted in a different global context, and highlighted lessons from it that might inform future research. In addition to reflections on unexpected events, challenges, and lessons learned, each chapter has also included a critical reflective conversation with a team member with firsthand knowledge about the study and the collaborating community. In so doing, this book attempts to provide information about the *speed bumps* that Fine (2007) describes as follows:

> the theoretical, methodological, and ethical struggles of researchers sitting with contradictory data and perspectives. These speed bumps are typically tucked away in the diaries of researchers or surface in quiet conversations among collaborators (Fine, 2007, p.464).

The book is limited in terms of the communities and contexts included yet hopes to provoke reflection and action among researchers who want to engage meaningfully with marginalized communities.

C. Logie, *Working with Excluded Populations in HIV*, Social Aspects of HIV 8,
https://doi.org/10.1007/978-3-030-77048-8_7

7.1 Key Principles When Working with Persons Categorized as Hard to Reach

7.1.1 Context Matters

The symbolic, material and relational dimensions of *context* matter and shape socio-cultural values and beliefs, access to resources and opportunities, and social capital. Researchers can examine how contexts shape risks and protective factors for HIV and other health issues, while also considering how research can be leveraged to enhance the value and dignity of marginalized communities, increase access to material resources and training, and foster respectful relationships and collective agency. In Chap. 2, which focused on research in Jamaica, we explored some of the assumptions made by myself, others, and the media about homophobic culture in Jamaica. We discussed false expectations that LGBT liberation would follow a similar patter to that observed in North America, involving large Pride demonstrations and marches, and the decriminalization of same sex sexual practices. When we listened carefully to the needs and priorities of LGBT persons locally, however, we learned about priorities for safety and nurturing and maintaining social relationships. This signalled the need to expand our perspectives to encompass alternative visions of LGBT futures, beyond North American aspirations. Here, it was key for ourselves as researchers to learn about micro-contextual meanings and expressions of pride, celebration, and intimate partnerships. Storytelling shed light on the local situation while also *recontextualizing* the larger social struggles engaged in by communities (De Fina, 2008).

In the Northwest Territories research project explored in Chap. 3, we discussed the importance of culturally grounded approaches that honour Indigenous ways of knowing and being. Important symbolic contexts described in the chapter included ceremony, land-based learning, and traditional crafts such as beading. Relational contexts included multi-generational learning with Elders and youth. Material contexts including logistic barriers (such as the weather) needed to be thoughtfully factored into study design. Land-based research approaches were central to the youth building relationships with themself and others. As Candice described it: “The land helps you to reflect on relationships because you’re in a relationship with the land. It helps you to reflect on all kinds of relationships, including your relationship with yourself, relationship with partners, with family, and within your community.” In this way we designed research to consider and take account of the wider physical and spiritual environment through both our methods and the epistemology.

Yasmeen explained how relational contexts and social capital were central to her ability to conduct community-based research with trans women in Chap. 4. Her long-standing relationships and service with communities of trans women resulted in knowing where and how to locate trans women to recruit for studies—and provided insight into designing studies that reflected the priorities of trans women themselves. Yet researchers with little personal or professional connection to trans women often expected her to leverage her personal connections, without investing the time and care to build their own relationships with trans communities. Yasmeen called for researchers to engage in relationship building with trans communities before designing a study based on the researcher's own interests: "There has to be some sort of relationship building before we can start to get involved or invite folks and say, 'OK, we are ready to do this research.'"

Veli described how she also did not have a hard time reaching LGBT community members in Eswatini for the research study we conducted there, because of her advocacy work and LGBT community engagement (see Chap. 5). The social capital generated by the community-based agency *The Rock of Hope* was so strong it readily facilitated research engagement: "When you heard "*Rock of Hope*" people wanted to participate." Yet there existed relational challenges, whereby LGBT persons at times felt less comfortable being interviewed by another LGBT person they might already know. This reflects the importance of moving beyond simply hiring LGBT persons to recruit participants and conduct data collection. Researchers should also consider the interpersonal dynamics within small and tight-knit LGBT communities (even in urban areas) and the need for careful planning and strategizing with community to mitigate confidentiality concerns.

Our work in Haiti, discussed in Chap. 6, revealed the interconnectedness between relational and material contexts. While initially conceptualized as an HIV prevention research project, *Famn an Aksyon Pou Sante Yo (FASY)* grew into becoming more than this. Peer health workers supported one other in facilitating weekly sessions and provided emotional and social support to participants by sharing their own personal stories of navigating survival, mental health, and relationship challenges. Participants described how through sharing these stories of struggle they experienced solidarity, including social support, happiness and feelings of unity. In addition to fostering social capital, peer health workers used monthly stipends to materially support family members, including building homes, paying school fees, and purchasing equipment to practice a trade, such as hair dressing. Years after the project, peer health workers continued to voluntarily provide literacy support to community members, reflecting relational contexts of social support that produced material benefits in increased reading comprehension.

Centering this relational perspective can also help to challenge the narrative that persons are hard to reach. With reference to the FASY project, CarolAnn described how the 'hard to reach' perspective individualizes issues rather than contextualizing the problem:

> It is the systems and the institutions for me that are the problem.... the narrative that we have about people who need help is part of the problem. This idea that if you need help, that there is something wrong with you... it is this very liberal idea of individualism that just creeps into everything that we do, that the ultimate goal is for all of us to be independent.

Our research with FASY revealed that community health workers, participants, families and wider communities benefited from the research project through its focus on building and sustaining relationships. Researchers should explore their own assumptions when they hear the term hard to reach, and whether we default to

the good things in trans women's lives. Lack of space for trans women of colour to discuss self-love and self-acceptance increased their interest in such strengths-focused research opportunities. Yasmeen also reflected on the reception she received when she presented TRANScending Love findings: "I can tell people there is hope, like despite what I have just told you about challenges facing trans people. . .There is hope, there is love and resilience. Sometimes I notice they also seem shocked. I think we can really get caught up in the academia part of it and forget the human side of it, at the end of the day these are human beings." Focusing on hope, feeling, goals and dreams can keep researchers connected with the shared humanity of people in their studies.

Chapter 5 discussed the impact that hope in the face of struggle had on the success of *The Rock of Hope*. The founder, Malume, had the hope and persistence to create this community agency founded on the premise that families and communities will support LGBT persons when provided with the right information and support. Malume's decision to promote joy and love, regardless of personal and professional challenges and hardship, established the blueprint for *The Rock of Hope* and other LGBT people in Eswatini. Underlying his outreach and educational work was Malume's belief that it could produce positive changes for the future. Veli described this hope for a better future: "One thing that Malume would always say is that with all the things that they were doing, it was not for them. It was with the understanding that there is a generation that is coming after and they should find things in a better space than they were before."

In Chap. 6, CarolAnn and I discussed the importance of researchers providing an opportunity for persons to see themselves reflected in the research process, and to celebrate communities. Our video to share HIV information and prevention messages was successful because it centered and represented the daily lives of people in the community, and people could see themselves in the bus, by the fire cooking, and watching the roosters wander around the yard[1]. These representations of daily life were the hook that brought people in to watch the HIV content. When we invited participants to bring family members to celebrate the end of the FASY project, entire communities came. Peer health workers, collaborators and participants themselves were hopeful and committed to the project's success. Throughout the research process, people gave us feedback—including on the day and time, facilitation, and refreshments—to help FASY improve and be as successful as possible. As CarolAnn described it, "They saw the importance of the work and wanted their community to be helped by it." Various components of hope emerged, including peer health workers meeting for years after the research project to help others learn literacy and the community wide celebration for participants. Together, these examples from studies across diverse contexts signal the potential for research to spark solidarity and hope in some of the most precarious environments.

[1]Famn an Aksyon Pou Sante Yo (FASY) video https://www.youtube.com/watch?v=YxjJ5dAtEmA.

7.1.3 Community Matters

A key finding across all the chapters in this book was the importance of research approaches that meaningfully engage with community members and provide a platform for people to identify and address their own priorities. Community-based research aims to amplify community members voices, priorities, and power in order to advance social change (Israel et al., 2003). Such an approach shifts what is considered legitimate knowledge by honouring lived experience, in turn reducing power imbalances between researchers and community-members participating in research. Research grounded in community collaborations and priorities offers sustainability, unanticipated benefits and offshoots, together with the promise of possibility. Community-based research aligns with Freire's conceptualization of praxis—or the unification of action with critical reflection that can spark critical consciousness, community organization, and transformation (Freire, 1972). At its heart, community-based research explores the issues that communities themselves identify as social problems and commits to leveraging research for social transformation.

Community-based research can also help develop new understandings of social phenomena that may be unchallenged or taken for granted. By characterizing values, meanings, and concerns among individual research participants, researchers can help to identify shared community goals and collective priorities for change. In turn, identifying shared priorities can generate collective identity and solidarity that builds community and shared responsibility. This caring and relational responsibility can be nurtured with proximal and distal others, signaling a stretching of socio-spatial relations (Darling, 2009) and caring practices across time and space ('caring-scapes') (Barnett & Land, 2007). Such a sense of community and caring can challenge the notion that people are hard to reach. As described in all the chapters in this book, community-embedded researchers did not believe that the people they worked with were hard to reach, as community connections and relationships identified and overcame participation barriers.

Earlier, when describing our research with LGBT young persons in Jamaica, Nicolette and I reflected on the finding that addressing harmful community norms, attitudes, and practices was perceived as more urgent than advocating for legal reform. Here, community connectedness and care are central to LGBT persons' survival. For instance, trans women in this context often supported one another's day-to-day wellbeing, and to do this they: "created tiny communities. They were able to bounce ideas off of each other and support one another." Participants also identified the importance of engaging beyond the LGBT community in Jamaica to effect long-lasting social change. For instance, despite ample evidence of the documented harms of criminalizing same sex practices, young LGBT people in Jamaica shared their local perspective that a focus on legal change would not be successful without also engaging in community-level transformation of hearts and minds.

As Candice discussed in the NWT, listening to community needs and preferences is key, even if this means following the community wish not to engage in research: "It's about building genuine relationships with communities and being ready to support communities in whatever way that they want, including to not engage with you" (Chap. 3). This statement also reflects the importance of researchers taking the time and commitment to build relationships with the communities that they want to engage with before embarking on a new study, and ensuring that research projects focus on community priorities. Communities' agency over their own research involvement should be recognized and respected, and this should take precedence over a researcher's interests and desire to design a particular study.

In Chap. 4 Yasmeen described the important role that research can play in connecting community members together. She described how trans women of colour may be isolated, and arts-based research could provide a place for community-building: "Just to be in that space, with African, Caribbean and Black trans women is to feel that there are more people like me. They're just not around as much in the community." She also described how the arts-based project described in the chapter built long-lasting connections with trans women and increased community trust in herself as a researcher and advocate.

In Chap. 5, Veli described how in the research process *The Rock of Hope* did not stop at recruiting potential participants from its current membership, but intentionally reached out to engage new persons both in the study as well as programming. In this way it widened its relationships with community, and this expansion created opportunities for more diverse voices to be included in the study: "We were trying to reach more people, to move beyond the circle of people that might already come into *The Rock of Hope*. It is important to include more voices." In this way, research was used as a tool to widen *The Rock of Hope's* community membership and reach to expand the range of voices listened to and included in LGBT research in Eswatini.

The *FASY* research project in Haiti, described in Chap. 6, shared the powerful lessons we learned about community while working in Leogane. CarolAnn described how "community relationship was privileged above everything else…when something happened, people came together in such an amazing way…that to me was transformational, both in terms of my own ideas about what it means to be in community as well as to see it in practice." This narrative also reflects how both CarolAnn and I were transformed by the research process to understand the responsibilities we had within the community. Much of the conflict we experienced in the research process was in part due to community collaborators' frustration with the lack of consistency, commitment, and humility among researchers more generally when they came to work in Haiti. Prolonged community engagement helped break down these barriers and was essential to our research success.

7.2 Recommendations for Future Research

Beyond context, hope, and the power of community, several other suggestions can be made for future research. These include the importance of cultural humility, the use of arts-based and other creative forms of storytelling, and the value of action-oriented research to benefit communities.

7.2.1 Cultural Humility

Throughout this book, researchers have been encouraged to practice cultural humility through self-reflection, community engagement, and ongoing learning in order to be flexible and prioritize community needs. Chapter 2 discussed how research projects may be limited in their ability to address socio-environmental inequities when working with LGBT persons. For instance, in Jamaica we could not bring about change in the socioeconomic, housing, and employment barriers experienced by LGBT persons—yet these were the key priorities in participants' lives. Continued funding was also challenging to acquire, leading to multi-year gaps in our research engagement. Recruiting LGBT participants in this project, and trans women in particular, required community engagement with peer researchers who were viewed as integral, valuable, informed team members who received sufficient financial compensation, research training, and support.

Chapter 3 discussed the importance of recognizing our own limitations—together with the limitations of an academic lens—in order to position ourselves as continuous learners. As Candice described: "we are always learning and we're always being humbled, because sometimes we're wrong and we need to own our mistakes. We need to allow ourselves that space to be uncomfortable. It's not easy sometimes, especially as an academic, to be uncomfortable and to feel like you don't know stuff." She also discussed how if researchers were not able to reach youth in the NWT, this might be due to a disconnect between research aims and the goals and priorities of young people themselves. This disconnect could, however, create the impetus to reflect and to work differently, by developing research plans collaboratively with community.

Similarly, in Chap. 4 Yasmeen described how she was "tired with the language of 'hard to reach'. It is the way that service providers and the researchers and the people who want to work with trans persons always seem to have probably not the right objective." Here, Yasmeen situates the problem in terms of the researchers' approach and intention, rather than potential participants. Yasmeen also draws attention to the histories of research exploitation experienced by trans communities that exacerbate feelings of vulnerability and misunderstanding. Her comments signal the need for researchers to reflect on their own personal biases and their relationships with trans women, and how these shape whether or not a researcher is perceived as trustworthy. Yasmeen explained that trans women should be recognized as experts: "Researchers and people coming in think they know what we need to know. They underestimate the knowledge that trans people have about themselves and their access to services in the community." Yasmeen also described the importance of being in touch with one's soul, to understand the underlying motivation for research and to interrogate what type of researcher one wants to be.

Chapter 5 described a participatory theatre project in Eswatini in which I felt the need to disrupt stigma when it emerged in the participatory theatre process, and the mixed emotions I then felt when enacting my power in this way. This reflects Fine's (2007) discussion of a *speed bump* and how processing the challenges encountered in the research process can provide insight into "the generative possibilities of our bodies and the meanings they bring with them" (McClelland, 2017, p. 7). My interventions with a colleague who misgendered Malume, a research participant who was openly homophobic, and in a participatory theatre skit that reproduced stigma, required awareness of my own values of social justice and my privilege and power as the research principal investigator. Cultural humility as a framework involves reflection on our emotions and positionality to provide us with insight into our privilege, and this reflection can shape our subsequent research interactions.

CarolAnn and I discussed in Chap. 6 the understandable wariness community collaborators had toward researchers who entered Haiti believing that they had more knowledge about the needs and priorities of the community than local people themselves. CarolAnn described the self-reflective stance that researchers need that is congruent with the concept of cultural humility: "Sometimes we need to think about our own stance and standpoint as it relates to these issues before we enter into spaces. I think that it is far easier to talk about people as a problem. . .than it is to talk about systems and institutions. Because we ourselves need to feel like we are doing what is right, so long as we have someone to blame. It is not easy taking on an institution or a system... And most of us do not have those skills." What then happens to our desire as researchers to be part of a solution, when the required solution is systemic and thus challenging, time consuming, requiring skills and expertise we may not have? A stance of cultural humility can help us to recognize and push beyond our comfort zone so as to privilege community interests, needs and priorities.

7.2.2 Arts-Based and Creative Storytelling Methods

Creative storytelling methods offer the chance to build empathy and understanding of our shared humanity. Participant narratives may point to counter-stories that identify and resist oppressive contexts, and document survival strategies (Solórzano & Yosso, 2002). Stories can also show everyday life experience as valuable and elevate experiential knowledge that may or may not align with scientific understanding.

In Chap. 3, Candice and I discussed the non-verbal approaches to communication that may be helpful with youth when discussing stigmatized topics such as sex. For instance, she described body-mapping (Lys, Gesink, Strike, & Larkin, 2018) as an alternative approach that may elicit different kinds of knowledge: "It is about engaging with the arts, using more than your words to explore things, to think about things—and sometimes to not think about things—and to just be in your body. It's a way of learning that is so versatile." She also discussed the potential of music in healing and stimulating dialogue in research processes, describing how "drumming can be connected to ceremony and to really important conversations". We also explored how Indigenous teachings can be adapted for different age groups to facilitate problem solving. The lessons embedded in storytelling and metaphors do not provide automatic answers, rather they can be used to guide decision making regarding complex issues including intimate relationships and safer sex practices. Researchers should consider engaging with multiple knowledge holders—including Elders, the land and animals—and sources of knowledge, such as dreams, traditional teachings, and ceremony.

Similarly, in Chap. 4 Yasmeen described the new possibilities that may emerge with the use of arts-based methods: "using an arts-based approach, it can bring out something in people that would not have come out in a focus group, for example, if we sat around and had pizza and asked persons to talk about self-love. But giving people something visually to work with, something that was really simple, it was so deep for a lot of people." She talked too about the importance of celebration. We produced a video series together, she produced a Trans Person of Colour (TPOC) cookbook, and we planned a red-carpet launch to celebrate the launch of the cookbook and video series. Celebration can challenge the depressing and pathologizing narratives that often surround trans women of colour. Celebration is both a source of motivation and hope that can be embraced in research. It can also provide a vision of future possibilities and new perspectives on oneself. Through pleasure and celebration, researchers can move beyond a focus on statistics and 'hard' knowledge to better understand hopes, goals and dreams. Adrienne Maree Brown's book *Pleasure Activism: The Politics of Feeling Good* (Brown, 2019) explores how building communities of care through activities such as sharing food can be a vehicle for collective healing and political resistance.

In Chap. 5, Veli discussed the power of theatre to inspire storytelling: "It is hard to just come across a person and tell them your life story and all of your experiences. But when people saw in the skits what LGBTI people experienced, somehow it made them relate a little bit more with us." In Eswatini, participatory theatre provided a way to share experiences of LGBT persons without asking people to share their personal stories—which could be both dangerous and exhausting. The theatre sparked conversation and dialogue in ways that produced empathy. Arts-based approaches can also be more appealing to people with little interest in the topic at hand. For instance, several participatory theatre participants shared how it was the specific kind of theatre that encouraged them to participate and which moved them emotionally, and how they would never have read a book on LGBT issues. Veli also highlighted how creative approaches that move beyond traditional knowledge dissemination platforms such as books, research articles, and conference presentations are more accessible to both LGBT and non-LGBT audiences in Eswatini.

7.2.3 Action-oriented Research to Benefit Communities

In Chap. 2, I reflected on the way in which the community partner in Jamaica took swift action to mobilize research findings so as to benefit LGBT persons and help build community engagement. Specifically, as there was shared ownership of data, the community partner used research findings to leverage funding to develop and implement trans support groups and training for clinic staff. As Nicolette described events: "we did not just sit down and look at this amazing data and say, well, we did this. We actually were and still are acting."

This action research focus was also present in Chap. 3. Candice had created FOXY as an action research project in order to have "a greater impact on the North than a dissertation that was going to sit on a shelf." FOXY aimed to positively impact the lives and sexual health of youth in the NWT. This focus and commitment was in part due to Candice's shared identity and lived experiences as a Northerner and Indigenous woman: "I struggled with a lot of things as a teenager and I wanted to do something to be who I needed when I was younger." Her continued research to evaluate and refine FOXY reflected a commitment to expanding opportunities for young people in the North. These include creating the Strengths, Masculinities and Sexual Health (SMASH) project through a community-engagement process to develop a program to engage boys and young men, and applying our LGBTQ research findings to make FOXY and SMASH programming more sexually and gender inclusive.

Yasmeen also focused on the importance of research in bringing about change in Chap. 4. She described how researchers need to ask themselves, "when the research is finished, how will this impact this particular population?" Researchers can work jointly with communities to engage in action-oriented inquiry. Similar to the way in which Nicolette described multi-phased research processes that could build lasting, trusting relationships with communities, Yasmeen explained how her research and programs built on one another. For instance, the trans women's cooking project was a spin-off from TRANScending Love, and several cooking project participants later took part in the trans women's resilience video series we produced[2]. Yasmeen's continued engagement and commitment to social change for trans communities strengthened community trust in her: "they know, again we are here, and we are going to make change in a different way."

In Chap. 5, Veli discussed the disconnect between community-based research and academic research. Stigma and discrimination constrained access to education and employment opportunities for LGBT persons in Eswatini and, subsequently, LGBT community members conducted their own grassroots research. This research however was not recognized by academic researchers, who often conducted studies that did not meaningfully engage LGBT persons or result in tangible benefits to the community. Veli invited researchers to consider how knowledge generation within

---

[2]Reflections of Trans Women of Colour: Love, Resilience, and Health - Series Introduction https://youtu.be/SGdh-VTzowU.

LGBT communities can benefit from the research process—as this could provide an incentive to participate. Expanding the ways in which findings are disseminated to communities can also increase the likelihood that research findings will be taken up in ways that create a positive social impact.

7.3 The Epistemology of Ignorance and the Concept of the Hard to Reach

An integrated approach to ignorance requires us to consider our agency in learning and acquiring knowledge (El Kassar, 2018). This integrated approach balances the need for knowledge acquisition; attitudes and beliefs about open-mindedness and curiosity; and recognition of the social and structural factors that reproduce false knowledge. As researchers, we need to consider all three of these factors and ask ourselves: what current and historical information are we missing with respect to a health issue and/or population; do we have an open-minded and curious mindset that will allow us to hear divergent perspectives and are we willing to adopt a new stance based on this information; and do we recognize the ways in which dominant power structures reproduce social and structural inequities in knowledge acquisition and dissemination?

In Chap. 2, an integrated approach to ignorance might mean that prior to beginning a research project, we as researchers need first to read literature from authors diverse in gender, ethno-racial identity, sexual orientation, gender identity, age and other lived experiences from the Caribbean region. We can consider the ways that racism, colonialism and histories of slavery shape the representation of Caribbean people and places in media and research, and the continued social, political, and economic effects. Taking the insights learned from these readings and considerations, we can reflect on our own openness to challenging our biases through acquiring new perspectives. For instance, I learned how young Jamaican LGBT persons' aspirations may differ from my own goals as a queer white woman from Canada.

It is also important to consider the perspectives that have been omitted from research. This reflects the *outwardlookingness* in relational perspectives of place that amplifies what can be learned from insider perspectives (Darling, 2009). When working in Jamaica, I first needed to unravel the ideas that decriminalization would be a priority for persons I worked with and that HIV was a key concern in their lives, in order to more properly explore the social practices of the communities. As Kippax et al. described: "the social practices people engage in 'co-constitute the world as it is' enabling communities to imagine, consider, discount, devise, adapt, and adopt particular HIV prevention strategies" (Kippax, Stephenson, Parker, & Aggleton, 2013, p. 1373). Researchers can reflect on historic and current power imbalances when centering the marginalised communities we are working with and for.

Applied to our research in the NWT in Chap. 3, this integrated approach to ignorance signalled the bi-directional relationship between knowledge acquisition and attitudes and beliefs. Embracing an attitude and belief system of cultural humility that encourages self-reflection and learning can help researchers to listen and learn about research needs and priorities. Cultural humility can also help researchers identify the social and structural factors that produce hegemonic knowledge systems (Tervalon & Murray-García, 1998; Yeager & Bauer-Wu, 2013). This requires continuous self-examination of our own assumptions, biases and values both as people and as researchers, and subsequently active work to transform inequitable power relationships, including in research processes. It also means developing a secure understanding of the role of non-Indigenous settler persons in the research process, histories of colonization and genocide, and the various protocols developed by Indigenous communities to guide research practices with Indigenous communities. The inward gaze of cultural humility, alongside an approach to culture as forward-looking, dynamic and complex, can help to dismantle stereotypes and other forms of false knowledge inherent within systems of ignorance. Adhering to Indigenous research protocols and recommendations can also provide accountability and a roadmap with which to challenge epistemologies of ignorance.

Chapter 4 discussed critical hopeful approaches using arts-based methods with trans women of colour. Alongside learning about trans communities and issues, reflective conversation with Yasmeen underscored the need to self-reflect on one's own intentions and motivations when working with trans women. This included considering whether or not one is a member of, or connected to, trans communities, and whose beliefs and interests have guided the development of research questions. It also includes learning about cisnormativity and cisgender privilege (Logie et al. 2019). Open mindedness and critical self-reflection are key for researchers to understand how the historic and current role of researchers and scientific communities in exploiting trans communities (re)produces research mistrust.

Chapter 5 explored the need to acquire knowledge about how to respectfully treat LGBT persons in Eswatini, and the importance of researchers understanding how and when to intervene to disrupt stigma. The participatory theatre aimed to provide knowledge on the lived experiences of LGBT persons, specifically regarding social and structural contexts of exclusion in family, healthcare, and public spaces. The theatre approach aimed to foster attitudes of open-mindedness, curiosity, and empathy, as well as to provide a chance to practice how to act in supportive and accepting ways toward LGBT persons in a rights-constrained context.

In Chap. 6, CarolAnn and I discussed researchers' perceptions of community needs and priorities—"when people come in with this idea that I know more about you than you know about yourself"—as a significant barrier to research engagement. Researchers should reconsider where and from whom they have acquired their existing knowledge and understanding (in this case, about internally displaced persons and Haitians) to consider whether it is grounded in lived experience. We identified important skills for researchers and practitioners to acquire—such as dismantling systemic and institutional barriers and inequities—to advance community priorities for social change. An open minded and curious stance can allow researchers to notice what outcomes are truly valuable for participants, such as the need to be respected in their community. Centering the community and our relationship with it can challenge dominant Western perspectives of knowledge, including perspectives where, as CarolAnn described, "the researcher is [. . .] seen as much more capable, intelligent", and the "idea that to be a good researcher is to be objective, to be removed from your 'subjects'". Instead, growing connections and relationship with communities can help us to better understand interdependence within communities and between researchers and those they seek to understand.

Together, an epistemologies of ignorance framing considers both knowledge and understanding, and attitudes and beliefs, through a social and structural lens (El Kassar, 2018; McGoey, 2012; Tuana, 2004). Elsewhere, Bowleg et al. propose the importance of applying an intersectionality framework to epistemologies of ignorance in order to recognize the interplay between multiple social identities (Bowleg et al., 2017). They describe how "intersectionality is ideally suited for 'identifying gaps in conventional logics', such as single-axis views of epistemic ignorance" (Bowleg et al., 2017, p. 578) and underscore the need for centering both history and social and structural contexts to overcome epistemic ignorance. When planning research with populations categorized as hard to reach, researchers can proactively reflect on and address epistemologies of ignorance regarding intersecting social categorizations (e.g., gender, race, age, income) and health issues (e.g., HIV, substance use) that may disrupt the research process.

7.4 Conclusion: Moving Beyond Vulnerability Toward an Enabling Environment

Similar to how the term 'hard to reach' has been critiqued as a vague catch-all descriptor, there have been calls to move beyond a focus on 'vulnerability' towards an analysis of structural inequities (e.g. Katz, Hardy, Firestone, Lofters, & Morton-Ninomiya, 2020; McLaren, Masuda, Smylie, & Zarowsky, 2020). A recent review of public health research found that the term vulnerable is too often used without explaining who is vulnerable, why, and what to (Katz et al., 2020). A focus on the structural production of inequities and power imbalances is largely absent from vulnerability narratives—also obscured are the persons who are considered *not* to be vulnerable. As a result, "authors imply that some populations are inherently vulnerable, compelling the reader to 'fill in the blanks' as to the root causes of their vulnerability. When readers fill in the blanks, some will turn to false and damaging ideas that permeate public health, policy and popular culture" (Katz et al., 2020, p. 606). Current vagueness surrounding the concept of vulnerability can inadvertently signal that individual level issues lie at the root of most health issues, or that structural issues are immutable.

Similar issues arise with the concept hard to reach. No person I interviewed across the community-based research projects described in this book considered the populations we worked with to be hard to reach—including LGBT persons in Eswatini and Jamaica, where same sex practices are criminalized, Indigenous youth in the Arctic, transgender women of colour in urban Canada, and internally displaced persons in post-earthquake Haiti. Instead, they discussed socio-historic contexts of research mistreatment and exploitation, colonization, and the disconnect between researchers and the communities they wish to work with. In future research, perhaps researchers could ask themselves the question: who is easy for me to reach, and what is it about their life situation that makes it easy for them to participate in the research as I have designed it? The answer may provide insight into who is being served by current research approaches, and their role in producing research that is hard to reach for some and not others (Katz et al., 2020).

Conversations about vulnerability and the challenges researchers encounter reaching people should never overshadow our focus on strengths, solidarity, hope and resilience among communities we are working with, and for. Kippax et al. (2013) provide a rich discussion of the potential ways for researchers to center persons labelled vulnerable and at high risk for HIV in ways that amplify their collective agency. A focus on vulnerability without concurrent attention to agency can be disempowering and individualizing, leading to limited "recognition or understanding of what connects people to each other, and what forms the stuff of their social and cultural lives" (Kippax et al., 2013, p. 1369). By framing persons as members of communities with collective agency—rather than individuals who are risky or vulnerable—researchers can explore our shared capacity to cope with and mitigate the harmful impacts of social and structural inequity. Understanding social norms and social practices can also provide insight into how communities cultivate connections, engage in collective action, and effect social change.

Community values and aspirations evolve, and community practices include experimentation and adaptation—making it difficult to produce a fixed blueprint for researchers to follow. This signals the importance of researchers listening and adapting to community processes and priorities. Researchers have a key role to play in producing enabling environments (Campbell & Cornish, 2012) that amplify the benefits of research for participants themselves and contribute to transforming power relations to produce more equitable living conditions. Throughout such a process, it is possible to reimagine research as a process that contributes to personal and collective *flourishing*, a process defined by the Merriam-Webster dictionary as growing "luxuriantly" and thriving[3].

[3]See https://www.merriam-webster.com/dictionary/flourish.

References

Barnett, C., & Land, D. (2007). Geographies of generosity: Beyond the 'moral turn.'. *Geoforum, 38*(6), 1065–1075.

Bowleg, L., del Río-González, A. M., Holt, S. L., Pérez, C., Massie, J. S., Mandell, J. E., & Boone, C. A. (2017). Intersectional epistemologies of ignorance: How behavioral and social science research shapes what we know, think we know, and don't know about U.S. black men's sexualities. *Journal of Sex Research, 54*(4–5), 577–603.

Brown, A. M. (2019). *Pleasure activism: The politics of feeling good.* Chico, California, USA: AK Press.

Campbell, C., & Cornish, F. (2012). How can community health programmes build enabling environments for transformative communication? Experiences from India and South Africa. *AIDS and Behavior, 16*(4), 847–857.

Darling, J. (2009). Thinking beyond place: The responsibilities of a relational spatial politics. *Geography Compass, 3*(5), 1938–1954.

De Fina, A. (2008). Who tells which story and why? Micro and macro contexts in narrative. *Text and Talk, 28*(3), 421–442.

Duncan-Andrade, E. M. R. (2009). Note to educators: Hope required when growing roses in concrete. *Harvard Educational Review, 79*(2), 184–194.

El Kassar, N. (2018). What ignorance really is. Examining the foundations of epistemology of ignorance. *Social Epistemology, 32*(5), 300–310.

Fine, M. (2007). Expanding the methodological imagination. *The Counseling Psychologist, 35*(3), 459–473.

Freire, P. (1972). *Pedagogy of the oppressed.* London, UK: Penguin Books.

Freire, P. (2004). *Pedagogy of indignation.* Boulder, Colorado, USA: Paradigm Publishers.

Freire, P. (2014). *Pedagogy of Hope: Reliving pedagogy of the oppressed.* New York, USA: Bloomsbury Publishing.

Israel, B. A., Schulz, A. J., Paker, E. A., Becker, A. B., Allen, A. J., & Guzman, J. R. (2003). Critical issues in developing and following community based participatory research principles. In *Community-ased participatory research for health.* San Francisco, CA: Jossey-Bass.

Katz, A. S., Hardy, B. J., Firestone, M., Lofters, A., & Morton-Ninomiya, M. E. (2020). Vagueness, power and public health: Use of 'vulnerable' in public health literature. *Critical Public Health, 30*(5), 601–611.

Kippax, S., Stephenson, N., Parker, R. G., & Aggleton, P. (2013). Between individual agency and structure in HIV prevention: Understanding the middle ground of social practice. *American Journal of Public Health, 103*(8), 1367–1375.

Logie, C. H., Lacombe-Duncan, A., Persad, Y., Ferguson, T. B., Yehdego, D. M., Ryan, S., Forrester, M., Moses, C., & Guta, A. (2019). The TRANScending love arts-based workshop to address self-acceptance and intersectional stigma among transgender women of color in Toronto, Canada: Findings from a qualitative implementation science study. *Transgender Health, 4*(1), 35–45.

Lys, C., Gesink, D., Strike, C., & Larkin, J. (2018). Body mapping as a youth sexual health intervention and data collection tool. *Journal of Qualitative Health Research, 28*(7), 1185–1198.

McClelland, S. I. (2017). Vulnerable listening: Possibilities and challenges of doing qualitative research. *Qualitative Psychology, 4*(3), 338–352.

Mcgoey, L. (2012). The logic of strategic ignorance. *British Journal of Sociology, 63*(3), 533–576.

McLaren, L., Masuda, J., Smylie, J., & Zarowsky, C. (2020). Unpacking vulnerability: Towards language that advances understanding and resolution of social inequities in public health. *Canadian Journal of Public Health, 111*(1), 1–3.

Shakur, T. (1999). *The rose that grew from concrete.* New York, USA: Pocket Books.

Solórzano, D. G., & Yosso, T. J. (2002). Critical race methodology: Counter-storytelling as an analytical framework for education research. *Qualitative Inquiry, 8*(1), 23–44.

Tervalon, M., & Murray-García, J. (1998). Cultural humility versus cultural competence: A critical distinction in defining physician training outcomes in multicultural education. *Journal of Health Care for the Poor and Underserved, 9*(2), 117–125.

Truth and Reconciliation Commission of Canada. (2015). *Canada's residential schools: Reconciliation – the final report of the truth and reconciliation commission of Canada.* Government of Canada.

Tuana, N. (2004). Coming to understand: Orgasm and the epistemology of ignorance. *Hypatia, 19* (1), 194–232.

Yeager, K. A., & Bauer-Wu, S. (2013). Cultural humility: Essential foundation for clinical researchers. *Applied Nursing Research: ANR, 26*(4), 251–256.

The manufacturer's authorised representative in the EU is Springer Nature Customer Service Centre GmbH, Europaplatz 3, 69115 Heidelberg, Germany. If you have any concerns regarding our products, please contact ProductSafety@springernature.com

Printed and bound by CPI Group (UK) Ltd, Croydon, CR0 4YY
30/09/2026
02225608-0016